_f_**P**

This book is dedicated above all to my mother, whose blossoming was
a continuous revelation and inspiration to me.

To all women who desire to transform themselves as they bloom into
their Second Spring and find grace, health, and youthful vitality in
their lives.

SECOND SPRING

===: DR. MAO'S :===

HUNDREDS *of* NATURAL SECRETS FOR WOMEN TO REVITALIZE AND REGENERATE AT ANY AGE

DR. MAOSHING NI

Free Press

New York   London   Toronto   Sydney

FREE PRESS
A Division of Simon & Schuster, Inc.
1230 Avenue of the Americas
New York, NY 10020

Manufactured in the United States of America

ISBN-13: 978-1-4165-9935-7

Contents

Introduction to
Your Second Spring

THIS IS A HEALTH BOOK FOR WOMEN to use at any age. You may be 35 and experiencing low energy, 50 and going through menopausal brain fog, or 75 and waking up each morning with arthritic pain. The good news is that, whatever your age, I will show you the ways to regenerate and revitalize. Welcome to your Second Spring.

I was inspired to write this book by watching my mother go through her middle years. Other women of her generation retired with their husbands and turned away from the world, but this was not her way. My mother energized and revitalized herself with Chinese medicine and refashioned her purpose in life. With her new freedom and the perspective of long experience, she turned her attention to interests that had developed gradually during her householding years. I looked on in admiration as she became a minister in her religious organization and turned her home into a temple to serve her community. In our family, my father, a doctor, was the public face of Chinese wisdom and tradition, while my mother, with all her character and dignity, was a modest woman who remained within the domestic sphere. Yet her personal transformation taught me more about human potential than I have learned from any other individual. It called into question the very concept of aging.

How do you feel about your age? Do you value yourself as you are? Your health at any point of your life depends on both your physical condition and your emotional attitudes about yourself and your life.

You can look and feel younger than your actual years and move through perimenopause, menopause, and beyond with grace, youthfulness, vitality, and health. Aging does not have to be a downhill slide. This book can help you achieve all this naturally—without drugs, hormone replacement, or invasive surgery. How? Through the wisdom of Chinese medicine, which is sensitive to all aspects of a woman's life cycle and understands that every phase affords opportunities to slow or reverse the aging process. This powerful tradition, integrated with Western medicine, can produce the optimum outcome for each individual.

On the emotional plane, Chinese tradition offers a paradigm completely different from the Western vision of midlife and aging. To the Chinese, this is the time when a woman truly comes into her own, when the distractions of the householding, childbearing, and child-rearing years wind down and her inner beauty emerges. A mature woman is a work of art crafted by her experiences and her own inner resources. She now refines her wisdom and finds traditional or inventive ways to make it useful in the world. Far from ceasing to grow, she embarks on a new path of self-realization.

Secrets to Our Success

At the Tao of Wellness, my brother Dr. Daoshing Ni and I, along with our team of associates, have helped thousands of women over the last 25 years. Our success is attributable to three factors. First, women have always been the cornerstone of Chinese society. From its inception thousands of years ago, Chinese medicine has developed a comprehensive specialty in women's health that is unrivaled in the world. Second, we draw on a profound knowledge base in women's health care, passed down through 38 continuous generations of doctors in our family. The third and most important ingredient is our patients' trust in our care and eagerness to do their part. Their willingness to inhabit new ideas and behaviors allows us to coach them through their Second Spring and help each one individually to reclaim her personal and sexual vigor.

Women's Cycles and Regeneration at Each Stage

Biologically, the ultimate purpose of human life, as with all living creatures on our planet, is reproduction, to pass on our genes from one generation to another. So, it is no surprise that, when you reach reproductive maturity, the organism's vitality starts to wane. This biological decline is programmed to begin in women around age 35. Of course, you can still live a long and fulfilling life, free from illness and disability, after that age, but you may benefit from some help with the changes your mind, body, and spirit will go through.

Menopause signifies the end of a woman's menstrual cycle and a major turning point in her life. Every woman's experience with it is unique. Most women stop menstruating between the ages of 48 and 52, but uncomfortable symptoms of perimenopause—the premenopausal period—can begin as early as 35 and last into menopause and beyond. Some women go through perimenopause in two to three years, but for others it lasts as long as 12 or 15 years. It may start with an irregular menstrual cycle along with an increase in premenstrual symptoms or PMS.

As you get closer to menopause and the cessation of your menstruation, new and more extreme effects appear, which can include hot flashes, insomnia, weight gain, and vaginal dryness. For the Chinese, menopause connotes the emptying of the conception channel and the depletion of the fertility essence, but it is also a time for generation of a new vital energy and the ripening of identity. Chinese medicine, attuned to every phase of a woman's reproductive cycle, uses methods tested by time and tradition to reinvigorate the body and mind at each stage.

The Second Spring: Rebirth at Midlife

With its intimate understanding of the female body, Chinese traditional medicine has always addressed the special needs of women throughout their lives, including conception, pregnancy, and childbearing as well as the onset of menopause. In fact, the wisdom about regeneration during menopause is so well recognized that there is a term for it:

Second Spring. A woman's Second Spring is the renaissance of youthful vitality and sexual vigor she enjoys when she takes advantage of the secrets and natural powers of Chinese medicine. When the body begins to undergo the changes that take her through perimenopause, menopause, and beyond, in the Chinese perspective this is a time for celebration in a woman's life, when she is possessed of wisdom and graceful beauty. This positive outlook on aging stands in stark contrast to the Western stigma against growing old. Second Spring describes an important opportunity for self-discovery and renewal in women's lives.

As you move toward menopause and beyond, your body produces less of the essential hormones, mainly estrogen and progesterone, that maintain the health of your bones and the elasticity of your blood vessels and skin. Of the many consequences, osteoporosis and heart disease are the two conditions most emphasized by the Western medical community, but quality-of-life issues such as wrinkled skin, lower vitality, and decreased libido can also become disheartening and affect other aspects of health. Emotionally, some Western women dread menopause as a loss of youth and fertility. To add to the physical challenges, in our youth-obsessed society menopause often means the beginning of an unspoken social devaluation for a woman.

But the truth is that no one need be a helpless victim to this phase of life. With the guidance of Chinese medicine, every woman can turn these changes into an empowering experience of rejuvenation.

The Western Medical Approach to Women's Health, Menopause, and Beyond

Women's health needs during and after menopause have been addressed quite differently by the Western medical establishment than by Eastern traditions and integrative medical approaches. In the mid-19th century, a menopausal woman suffering hot flashes, depression, and painful, irregular periods would sometimes undergo a *hysterectomy*—surgical removal of the uterus—on the misconception that this organ was the source of women's physical and mental problems. Although doctors' understanding of these matters changed, the rate of hysterectomies remained high, and a large percentage of the operations were later found to be unnecessary.

In the past 40 years, Western medicine's solution for menopause has been the use of hormone replacement therapy (HRT). Its greatest popularizer was a gynecologist named Robert Wilson, whose outlook revealed more than a little sexism and ageism. He called menopause a "living decay." Supplemental estrogen, he and others insisted, was the ultimate answer.

Belief in the benefits of long-term HRT became entrenched in the medical community and among women of menopausal age. Doctors who delved into the issue more closely, however, were often surprised to learn how thin the evidence really was. Finally, in 2002, after decades of routine hormone replacement therapy, the landmark Women's Health Initiative made front-page headlines all over the country, and the news wasn't good. The study proved conclusively that HRT with a common blend of estrogen and progestin, when used for more than four years, increased women's risk of breast cancer, heart disease, stroke, and blood clots. Further studies confirmed that the risks of long-term HRT outweigh the benefits.

Chinese medicine has long recognized that the body is fully capable of regenerating and that supporting the natural production of all the essential hormones through natural means is safe, effective, and sustainable over a woman's lifetime. In other words, teach your body to rejuvenate itself instead of replacing your body's natural abilities.

Start Now to Create Your Personal Second Spring

It's important to get ready for the changes ahead. By making certain lifestyle, dietary, and mental adaptations now, you can avoid unnecessary suffering now and down the road. For instance, perimenopause may begin two years earlier in a woman who smokes than in one who doesn't. So don't be a victim of your own inaction—start preparing for your Second Spring right away. The advice in this book takes minimal effort to implement, but your rewards will be substantial.

In this guide, you will learn why Second Spring is a time of rebirth and renewal and how you, too, can experience a smooth transition, empowered by natural, time-honored practices. In the chapters that follow, you will learn many tips relating to diet, herbal therapy, exercises, meditation practices, acupressure, beauty, and lifestyle that will aid you in your personal Second Spring. You will find your own path to becoming young, sexy, and revitalized, and begin to blossom into a new phase of your life.

Your future is in your hands, and by happy coincidence, so is this book. Let me invite you to make the most of both. May you live long, live strong, and live happy.

CHAPTER 1

Ageless Beauty

I'VE CHOSEN TO BEGIN THIS BOOK with a chapter on beauty for a simple reason: We tend to notice the face and outward appearance first. What we often forget is that imbalances in a person's life and within her being show up on her face and skin. Your appearance reflects who you are—your physical health, emotions, and spirit. The tips given in this chapter will guide you in beautifying your inner and outer self.

Skin Aging and Thinning Hair are Not Inevitable

Asian women's secrets to baby-soft skin include Chinese botanicals, beauty foods, acupuncture, massage, and natural skin treatments along with meditation, facial exercise, and detoxification techniques. You can use them to obtain a glowing complexion and a smooth, well-toned face.

Your skin is the largest organ of your body. It acts as a protective fortress against the outside, barring bacteria, viruses, and fungi from invading; it keeps heat and moisture inside; and it expresses your emotional and nervous states via its color, texture, and condition. Your skin has three layers: the epidermis, dermis, and subcutaneous, each with specific functions and properties.

Epidermis—the outermost layer. This is the protective layer of your skin. When damaged—by sunburn, for example—it sheds and peels off, and new skin cells replace the old ones. Within the epidermis is the basal cell layer, which produces melanin, the substance that gives your skin color and protects against the sun's ultraviolet rays. It is responsible for your nice tan but can also produce undesirable blotches, freckles, and age spots. When the basal cell layer is extremely overstressed it can even become cancerous. This chapter provides natural techniques to help cleanse and renew your epidermis.

Dermis—the sandwich layer. The middle layer, or dermis, is perhaps the most important one. It contains blood vessels, nerve endings, and the cells that produce elastin and collagen, proteins that lend skin its resiliency. The circulation of blood through this layer brings nutrients to the skin and carries away waste. As a woman ages, collagen production decreases, and by midlife it is down about 20 percent. Declining secretions from the oil glands, along with free radical damage from diet, environment, and stress all act to thin the dermis. When this layer is not functioning optimally, dryness and wrinkles appear. Acupuncture, facial massage, herbs, and supplements can increase collagen and elastin production and tone the skin naturally.

Subcutaneous—the fatty layer. Just beneath the dermis, this layer serves as padding between the skin and the connective tissue of the muscles. it also insulates to preserve body heat. The subcutaneous contains deeper blood vessels, sensory and motor nerves, and a nutrient reservoir for the skin's upper layers. In women, this fatty tissue gives the softer angles and attractive curves on face and body. Dietary and nutritional therapies using food items as common as apple cider vinegar and as unusual as jellyfish can prevent thinning of the subcutaneous layer, as we will see later in the chapter.

Underneath the three layers of your skin are the connective tissues—muscles, tendons, and ligaments. No other animal has evolved as complex a set of facial muscles as humans have. The muscles of the face and neck are all joined together in a crisscross, quiltlike fashion. Facial exercises in this chapter will allow you to tone and shape your face as you would your body to attain a healthy, youthful look.

Close to 40 percent of women above 50 experience hair loss, sometimes beginning as early as their mid-30s. This is mainly due to changing hormonal balance, specifically the conversion of estrogen into excess androgen. If you are using estrogen replacement therapy and you notice hair loss, talk to your doctor about getting off the hormone safely. Never simply stop taking a medication without consulting your physician. Sometimes hair loss can result from thyroid dysfunction or overproduction of the hormone DHT. Of course, trauma, stress, poor nutrition, and bad circulation can all contribute to hair loss. Tips in this chapter show how to balance your hormones and regrow your hair.

Three Treasures are the Foundation of the Second Spring

In Taoist philosophy, the three components of a whole person consist of *shen*, *qi*, and *jing*—spirit, energy, and essence, respectively. They are also called the three treasures. When you have an abundance of each treasure and a healthy balance among them, beauty and vitality are the natural results. Restoring and cultivating the three treasures has been the underpinning of anti-aging science in the Taoist tradition for over five millennia.

Any discussion of beauty and health must start with the first of the three treasures—*shen*, or *spirit*. The spirit is the guiding force of our being and our life. It encompasses our conscious and unconscious minds. When the spirit is confused or distressed, it is expressed as distortion and tension in your face and elsewhere in your body. Clarity of spirit reflects externally as a smooth complexion and a contented, relaxed face with minimal lines. Western surgery would have you nip and tuck your way to a younger you, but if you fail to address your spirit and emotional well-being, this is at best temporary and often futile. With meditations and visualizations you can develop and continually refine your spirit.

The second of the three treasures, *qi*, or *energy*, defines the quality of your life experience. Without adequate energy, organ systems cannot operate properly and the cells become sluggish, leading to frequent breakdowns or disease. Likewise, your spiritual state will directly influence your energy. Negativity represses and blocks, while positive spiritual states uplift and fuel you. Energy comes from many sources, chiefly food, air, and sleep. When the sources are impure or contaminated, as with toxins in food or pollution in the environment, the energy derived is unsuitable for revitalizing your body's *qi*. Chinese herbs, acupressure, and qi gong practices promote optimal organ function and boost energy.

The natural chemicals Western science calls hormones represent aspects of *jing*, or *essence*, the third treasure. These substances are critical in the growth, development, and renewal of the skin. Additionally, *jing* is your genetic potential. Whatever your genetics, you can take steps to help your body express good genes and inhibit the action of bad genes. For instance, a fair-skinned woman will need extra sun protection compared to someone with dark skin, because, genetically, her skin is more vulnerable to damage. Essence can be nurtured through herbs, nutritional supplements, and nourishing foods.

Ensuring joyful spirit, abundant energy, and enduring essence is the foundation of health and beauty. But you must also eliminate toxins in the body that hamper your efforts to rejuvenate your skin. My integrative detoxification techniques employing nutritional, supplemental, and herbal protocols, coupled with topical cleansing and exfoliation, can usher you toward a fresh, new beginning in beauty and energy.

I invite you to explore the natural remedies, techniques, and practices that follow to help you attain ageless beauty.

Your skin
reflects your life

Beauty is more than skin deep, but your skin does reflect your health and your experience. The skin is constantly breathing, changing, and working to renew itself. All three layers of your skin—epidermal, dermal, and subcutaneous—function together to protect you, nourish you, and regulate the temperature of your body. Many factors affect the quality of your skin, ranging from diet and mood to environment and lifestyle. For example, a poor diet lacking nutrients is a recipe for bad, unhealthy skin. Alternatively, studies show that a nutritious diet—particularly of leafy greens and dried plums—can have a protective effect against wrinkling. Depression, anxiety, and stress create tension in your skin, particularly on the face and causes uneven blotches and lines. Sun damage and dry, cold, or windy weather rob the skin of vital moisture and circulation, leading to prematurely older-looking skin. Finally, smoking, excessive alcohol use, and lack of sleep all show up on your skin, reflecting your excesses like signed confessions.

Antiwrinkle Acupuncture

One of the secrets of Chinese women's youthful looks is the acupuncture face-lift. For centuries, the empresses and concubines of China's imperial palace used specialized techniques to erase fine lines and prevent wrinkles. Facial acupuncture is not a surgical procedure, but steadily improves muscle and skin tone in the face and slows the effects of gravity. Studies show that acupuncture increases blood flow in the tiny capillaries of the skin and muscles and stimulates collagen production in the dermis layer, increasing skin elasticity. The course is typically 10 to 12 treatments over two or three months, combined with nutritional and herbal supplements, which you will find in the next section. Be sure to work with practitioners who are specially trained in acupuncture for the face. Typical points include GB-14 to relax the forehead, Yintang to ease furrowing between the brows, Taiyang to get rid of crow's-feet around the corner of the eyes, and LI-20 and ST-3 for diminishing smile lines. You can also do acupressure on yourself, as shown in the next tip.

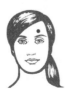

GB-14   LI-20   ST-3   Taiyung   Yintang

Do-it-yourself "face-lift"

Some wrinkles can be distressing signs of aging. You see them on the surface, but to address them, you need to look deeper. The middle layer of the skin, or dermis, supports the epidermal outer layer with nutrients from the blood and produces two crucial elements, collagen and elastin—proteins that support the connective tissue and give resilience to the skin. Like acupuncture, acupressure, the art of acupuncture without needles, can give you a nonsurgical face-lift, by toning facial muscles and stimulating natural production and deposit of collagen in the skin. You can learn to do acupressure on yourself. Simply press firmly with your fingers, working your way methodically along the wrinkle line, and your body will respond with increased circulation and nutrient delivery. Do this in the morning and at night for beautiful skin tone well into your late years. For specific points, please refer to previous tip.

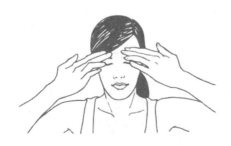

Gymnastics for your face

To tone up your facial muscles, give them a workout!
Do these exercises twice a day, five repetitions apiece:

1) Raise your eyebrows as high as you can—strain for it—and then relax them.

2) Try to move your nose from side to side.

3) Inflate your cheeks as though you're blowing up a balloon, then relax.

4) Open your mouth as wide as it can go, then stick out your tongue as far as you can. Hold for five seconds.

After all that hard work, your face deserves a massage. Stroke the whole face with a circular motion to warm it up. Then with the thumb and first finger of both of your hands pinch five times along your eyebrow line, from inside to outside. Press along both sides of the nose, where it meets the cheeks, from top to bottom, five times. Press the area around the outside of the mouth five times. Gently pat your cheeks with your fingers to stimulate the side of your face. Press the forehead lines between your eyebrows five times along each line. Now press the edges of the eye orbit, pushing gently above the eye and under its lower rim. Finish the massage with another round of circular strokes all over the face.

 1   2   3   4

Skin secrets
of Chinese courtesans

The outermost layer of the skin regularly renews itself
by shedding old cells and replacing them with new ones.
By hastening the shedding process, you can immediately
diminish the appearance of fine lines and wrinkles. Costly
medical procedures such as dermabrasion, chemical
peel, and various laser therapies also do this, but they can
produce redness and irritation lasting for days afterwards.
There are gentler ways to renew your skin with products
from nature. For centuries, Chinese imperial courtesans
used seaweed, kelp, pearl powder, dried plum, winter
melon seed, persimmon leaf, and cane sugar—natural
exfoliation and polishing agents that loosen and strip
dead skin cells off evenly. Most of these ingredients are
available in health food stores and Chinese groceries.
Make a mask with these natural ingredients listed above,
in any combination. Simply moisten with water and place
in a blender with aloe vera gel or egg white to make a
paste. Scrub gently with a wet loofah sponge, using small
circular motions, until face and neck are thoroughly ex-
foliated. Leave the mask on for 10 minutes, then wash off.
Avoid getting in your eyes.

Rich is poor
. . . nutrition

In Chinese medicine, rich foods like dairy, meat, fats, sweets, and alcohol are said to cause phlegm and dampness in the body. I have observed this phenomenon consistently in my patients: When they consume excessive amounts of these things, they develop a variety of symptoms such as sinus and chest congestion, postnasal drip, a sensation of heaviness, joint pain and stiffness, abdominal bloating, gas, loose bowel movements, high cholesterol, brain fog, fatigue, depression, and, of course, obesity. Most people don't have to completely eliminate the phlegm- and dampness-inducing foods; if you simply cut down on the quantity and frequency of consumption, you will improve how you feel overall. And you'll also lighten both your weight and your mood.

Filtered Water: Drink up!

Life originated in water, our bodies are 60 to 70 percent water, and this precious fluid is key to good health at every age. But as we get on in years, the body's organs weaken and the kidneys can't hold water the way they used to. Without sufficient fluid, toxins accumulate in the body, slowing down organ function and causing premature aging. Most women simply don't take in enough water, even though they're losing it more rapidly than when they were younger. It's easy to develop a "drinking habit"—the good kind! I suggest you get two large, rigid thermos bottles with a 20-ounce capacity. Fill them with water, take one along with you during the day to drink at work or as you run errands, and when you come home, drink the other one.

You will want to be sure you are drinking the purest water. Many studies have shown that tap water is filled with contaminants, antibiotics, and a number of other unhealthy substances. Consider investing in a good quality carbon-based filter for your tap water. If you find that plain water is just too plain, add a slice of lime or lemon, or make green or mint tea.

Pear away wrinkles and dark circles

If you don't like those lines you see when you look at your face in the mirror, have some *Asian pear*, a tasty fruit that's filled with vitamin C and, like dried plums, a good source of copper. These antioxidant nutrients help protect you from the ravages of free radicals, which alter the chemical structure of your cells. When free radicals damage enough cells, especially in the skin, signs of aging soon appear. Copper is an essential component of super-oxide dismutase (SOD), an enzyme that attacks these harmful agents when they enter the body via air pollution and other toxins. Pears, particularly the Asian (or Fuji) variety, juicy and with a crunchy texture, are prized by Chinese herbalists as a way to eliminate dark circles under the eyes. They also use pears to cure laryngitis and treat coughs and sore throats. In addition to its healing and skin-preserving properties, pear contains plenty of fiber, which lowers cholesterol and contributes to regularity, important for a clear complexion.

When toxins go, beauty glows

Toxins ranging from environmental pollution to pesticides and preservatives in our food hasten the aging process of our skin. The skin is the body's largest elimination organ, but it is often overloaded and unable to expel the toxins. Adding insult to injury, many of today's personal care and cosmetic products contain carcinogenic chemicals that are absorbed into the skin. A fundamental principle of Chinese medicine is that you help the body cleanse itself so that toxins do not cause internal imbalance, which shows up on your skin as premature aging signs.

Certain foods are traditionally used to help your body eliminate toxins: seaweed, bitter melon, Chinese cucumber, burdock, lotus root, and ginger. Try to include one of these in your diet every day. Herbs that detoxify the system can be found in a formula called Internal Cleanse, available in most Chinese herb shops. It contains plant substances such as dandelion, chrysanthemum, peppermint, white mulberry, and licorice, which assist and support healthy liver and gall bladder function. These organs play a role in detoxification and elimination so that the skin is not overburdened in its vital task. Follow the directions on the cleansing formula you buy, as each is slightly different.

Apple cider vinegar:
drink it and dab it

A traditional remedy to cure various digestive disorders, *apple cider vinegar* is also an effective toner for your skin. Taken internally, it supports liver detoxification, normalizes digestive juices, and reduces intestinal bloating. Mix 1 tablespoon of organic vinegar—be sure it's the apple cider kind—with 12 ounces of warm water, and drink in the morning on empty stomach. Add a little honey if the taste is too strong. The malic acid in vinegar, a natural alpha-hydroxy acid, can also be used externally to help renew your skin by ridding the epidermis of dead skin cells. Dilute one part cider vinegar in two parts distilled water. After cleansing your skin as you usually do, apply the diluted vinegar solution with a cotton pad to your face and neck. Follow with moisturizing lotion.

Out, out,
damned age spots!

Age spots, sun spots, liver spots, freckles, and skin blotches inhabit the topmost layer of your skin, also called the *basal cell layer*. The hormone melanin gives you your natural skin tone and protects you from sun exposure, but when too much pigment is produced, these undesirable discolorations can result. In severe cases a form of skin cancer, *basal cell carcinoma*, can occur.

Western medicine uses lasers, liquid nitrogen, and dermabrasion to remove these discolorations. Traditional Chinese practice has always recognized that one must treat the underlying mechanism of excess pigment deposit. Melanin is produced in response to hormonal signals from the kidney organ network, thus these skin spots that appear around menopause reflect a kidney imbalance. The quickest way to restore healthy kidney function is with diet, herbs, and nutritional supplements. Eat extra servings of black beans, sesame seeds, and mulberry, rich in antioxidants like saponin, lignan, and anthocyanin. Chinese herbalists offer formulas with herbs like Chinese yam, Asian cornelian fruit, and goji or lycium berry. Additional helpful supplements include alpha-lipoic acid, acetyl-L-carnitine, and quercetin, which help skin regenerate and remove pigment deposits; DMAE (dimethyl-amino-ethanol), a nutrient found in anchovies and sardines, is a powerful membrane stabilizer that reverses age spots on the skin.

Beauty food
for supple skin

The skin is merely the outer covering of the vast network of connective tissue that keeps all our organs intact and bones connected. Skin contains proteins, such as elastin and collagen, that work to maintain its structure and pliability. As you get older and closer to menopause, estrogen and progesterone decrease, contributing to a decline in proteins in the epidermis, which lessens skin elasticity. In China, it was a tradition in the imperial courts for the empress to pass down to the princesses her skin-beautifying recipes and preparations. The ingredients tended to be exotic, expensive foods such as bird's nest, shark's fin, and sea cucumber. While the first two are extremely hard to come by, sea cucumber—actually an animal—is fairly accessible. A relative of the starfish, sea cucumber contains essential amino acids that are the building blocks of collagen and elastin, and is available dried in Chinese food stores, ready to be used in soups. It is also available in supplement form. A typical dosage is 700 to 1,000 mg daily. Other foods for skin health from the imperial court beauty recipes include cherries, peanuts, black soybeans, walnuts, and jujube dates.

Nature's gentle skin peel

Skin peels are probably the fastest way to look younger. Cosmetic dermatologists generally use prescription agents such as Retin-A, high-concentration glycolic acid, and harsh chemicals for peels. While these procedures do produce a smooth skin finish and lessen lines, they also strip away the skin's protective layer and can increase your susceptibility to sun damage, skin aging, and skin cancer. The FDA warns that high concentration of various skin-peel agents may thin the skin. You can make simple at-home skin peels right out of your refrigerator. Use vegetables and fruits containing natural acids: eggplant, tomatoes, grapefruit, pineapple. Cut in thin slices or squares and place on your face and neck, covering the skin thoroughly; leave on for 20 minutes, then remove the pieces from your face and wash with warm water. Your face will look red for a few minutes, but this should clear up shortly. Use a natural moisturizer after you are finished. Natural peels are easy to do and, in time, will give you the smooth skin you are looking for.

Orange aid
for the complexion

Citrus is considered a superfood for healthy skin. Many studies have confirmed the healing properties of oranges, attributed to a wide variety of phytonutrients that function as antioxidants. These include flavanones, anthocyanins, polyphenols, and vitamin C. One type of flavanone specific to oranges, hesperidin, has anti-inflammatory properties and lowers blood pressure and cholesterol. Tangerine peels are traditionally used in Chinese medicine to improve digestive function and circulation. According to a study published in the Journal of Agricultural and Food Chemistry, compounds in the orange peel called *polymethoxylated flavones* (PMFs), have the potential to lower cholesterol more effectively than some prescription drugs—without the side effects.

Give your breasts a natural lift

Gravity affects your breasts as you age. Many women turn to quick-fix options like breast implants or breast-lifting surgery, but gravity will continue to act on the "improved" bust as well. The female breast is an organ made up mostly of fat—but keep in mind that it is held up ultimately by the muscles underneath (the pectoralis muscles, or pecs) and some muscles between the ribs as well. To help strengthen the pectoralis muscles, hold a 2-pound weight in each hand, extend your arms sideways, and move them in small circles, rotating toward the back. After 10 small circles, gradually widen the circles. Do 3 sets of 10 repetitions, with a little break in between, twice a day. Work your way up to 5-pound weights over time. Push-ups are another helpful exercise. You may want to start with girl's push-ups—on your knees—10 push-ups at a time. As you get stronger, graduate to true push-ups, 3 sets of 10, twice a day. The farther apart your arms, the better the effects. No matter what age you are, this is a great exercise for building upper body, arm, and core strength.

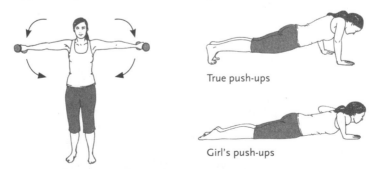

True push-ups

Girl's push-ups

Remedy rosacea
nature's way

A chronic skin problem that reddens the forehead, nose, cheek, and sometimes the chin, *rosacea* sometimes shows up at midlife. Scientists believe there may be a genetic predisposition to the condition, and some recent research suggests that mites that naturally occur on human skin are more abundant in people with rosacea. Outbreaks can be triggered by many things, including temperature extremes, sunlight, alcohol, caffeine, spicy foods, and certain medications. To treat rosacea, I focus on soothing the spirit, clearing heat, and removing blockages in the skin with natural remedies. A cucumber mask is perfect for this. Shave the skin off the fresh cucumber and puree the flesh in a blender with one egg white. Coat your face with this mixture and leave it on for 30 minutes. Wash off with cold water. Used daily, this mask will produce definite improvement within a month. Along with this, try taking B-complex vitamins, digestive enzymes, and 1,000 IUs of vitamin E every day.

Pretty
as a peach

Perhaps for its wealth of beneficial attributes, the peach symbolizes fertility and longevity in Chinese culture. Peaches are excellent sources of potassium and vitamins A and C. They have diuretic and mild laxative properties, help with digestion, and add color to the complexion. In fact, peaches have been used in beauty tonics throughout Chinese history. Beauty and longevity—how can you resist the power of the peach? In addition, peach leaf is anti-parasitic, and the fatty acids in peach kernel help regulate circulation, tame high blood pressure, and promote healthy metabolism. These are typically taken as an herbal tea, one to two cups per day. One beauty recipe calls for eating baked peaches with honey and lavender: Drizzle the halved peaches with honey, sprinkle with lemon zest and sprigs of fresh lavender, and bake for 30 minutes. A healthful, beautifying treat!

Sun therapy
for skin disorders

The human body needs sunlight to produce vitamin D, a fat-soluble vitamin crucial to the absorption of calcium and the building of healthy bones and teeth. It also plays an important role in preventing breast cancer, keeping blood pressure in check, lowering cholesterol, and—as Western research finally learned—maintaining healthy skin. That is why in China, over the ages, sunlight has been used to help skin problems like acne, eczema, and psoriasis. I often tell my patients with these skin conditions to lie in the sun for 20 minutes daily, using no sun block, before 10 a.m. or after 3 p.m. It usually takes about two to four weeks to see favorable results. For your face, limit your sun exposure to fifteen minutes. If you are treating skin problems elsewhere on your body, be sure to wear sunglasses and a wide-brimmed hat to protect your eyes and face. Drink a glass of water before and after each sun therapy session.

Wash your face
with yogurt

A favorite traditional tonic for healthy skin, yogurt contains *lactic acid*, a naturally occurring alpha hydroxy acid that is superb for creating a smooth skin texture. It is especially beneficial for those with sensitive skin that cannot tolerate commercial alpha-hydroxy acid preparations. Yogurt gently peels off the dead skin layer, rejuvenating the epidermis beneath. Over time, it can also lighten spots and even out a patchy skin tone. Apply organic plain yogurt like a cream to your freshly washed face, leave on for 15 minutes, then wash off. Finish up with a moisturizer. For even better results, steam your face with a facial steamer before rubbing the yogurt onto your skin. Always use cold water to wash off the yogurt and, if necessary, apply a cold pack for 10 minutes to reduce redness.

Jellyfish: a delicacy
for smooth skin

With its beautiful, luminescent membranes that resemble parachutes floating amid the ocean waves, a jellyfish is mesmerizing to look at. Few Westerners venture to eat jellyfish, but Asian women consider it a delicacy and a top nutrient for beautiful skin. Jellyfish is full of a calcium-binding photoprotein called *aequorin* that helps keep cells healthy and structurally strong. Studies show that aequorin slows aging and prolongs the life of cells. Supplements containing these proteins have been found to reduce cell death by up to 50 percent. Jellyfish is also recommended in Chinese medicine to restore elasticity to blood vessels in patients with hypertension. As we age, our own protective calcium-binding proteins become depleted, and jellyfish can help restore our supply. If you're not ready to try some jellyfish at an Asian restaurant, you can take its age-defying protein in supplement form. Aequorin is found in select health food stores and online.

Sesame
for skin and hair

Women of ancient Babylon would eat halva, a mixture of honey and sesame seeds, to extend youth and beauty; Roman soldiers ate the same blend for vigor and power. Sesame contains a rich supply of copper, manganese, calcium, magnesium, iron, phosphorous, zinc, and vitamins B and E, which are all essential for skin and hair health. More important, it possesses phytoestrogens called *sasamin* and *sesamolin*, which have antioxidant, anticancer, and cholesterol-lowering properties. It is no surprise that sesame is a favorite food among Chinese women for promoting beautiful hair and skin, long recognized for its nourishing virtues. You can toss the toasted seeds into rice dishes, use sesame butter in hummus, or drizzle tahini (crushed sesame seeds) on baked dishes or salads—delicious ways to get your fill of this wondrous little seed.

Brush away
bad hair days

A famous Chinese empress had a full head of beautiful black hair at the end of her long life. She reputedly had her scalp and hair brushed 500 strokes by her personal attendant upon rising and before retiring each day. Few women have the luxury of an assistant to brush their hair and massage their scalp daily, but you can more easily have healthy hair. Using a brush made with natural bristles or wood—not plastic, which generates undesirable static electricity—gently stroke your scalp as you brush your hair, stimulating the hair follicles and increasing the microcapillary circulation that feeds them nutrients. In addition, brushing full strokes from the head down to the tips will spread the scalp's natural oils along the hair shaft for shiny, supple hair. Studies show steady massage and brushing over time stems hair loss, promotes hair growth, and generally improves hair quality.

Natural treats for
shiny, healthy hair

Try massaging your scalp with fresh ginger juice to prevent hair thinning and loss. Squeeze a 1-inch chunk of ginger root in a garlic press to yield a small amount of juice. Drip fresh ginger juice on part of scalp with thinning hair with a dropper. Another option is to dissolve 1/2 teaspoon ginger powder in 1 tablespoon of hot water, and apply as described above. Leave it on for 15 to 20 minutes and then rinse it out—or leave it on overnight to stimulate the hair follicles. For shiny hair, once a week, mash a ripe avocado, massage it into your hair and scalp, and leave it on for 1 to 2 hours. If you wish to dye your hair, choose a natural colorant: Henna is excellent for shades of light brown and red; coffee or black tea may be used by brunettes; chamomile and lemon juice will color light hair. The Chinese use herbs to reverse graying: *Shou wu* or *fo-ti*, a hair-nurturing supplement available in Asian pharmacies, is derived from natural plant sources and has many other tonic properties. Your dietary choices can also help your hair. Eat plenty of black beans, black sesame seeds, and walnuts.

Oils you eat
shine your hair

Dryness or brittleness in skin, hair, eyes, and other parts of the body is common among women at midlife, due to the drop in estrogen in their bodies. But it is not inevitable. Natural remedies can prevent or reverse the loss of luster and suppleness. Start by making sure you have an abundance of good oils in your diet, the poly- and mono-unsaturated oils, which include flaxseed, sesame, olive, and virgin coconut oil, all excellent with salad greens. Their essential fatty acids and omega-rich nutrients keep your skin and hair well lubed. Also, eat up to two small hand-fuls of nut and seed combinations—pine nuts, hazelnuts, walnuts, sunflower seeds—every day between meals. Another excellent food is avocado, which is not only rich in good fats but also abundant in *glutathione*, the antioxi-dant compound that helps reverse premature aging of cells. Half an avocado a day provides you with abundant nutrients beneficial to your hair. However, be sure not to eat more than advised; although these foods contain the good types of fats, overeating them will make you gain weight.

CHAPTER 2
Find Your Ideal Weight

OVER THE YEARS, many of my female patients have come to me complaining that they keep gaining weight, especially around the waist, even though they eat the same amount of calories or less. They feel constantly bloated and sluggish, and they no longer fit into their clothes. This weight gain is not only emotionally frustrating, it can also have dire health consequences, such as increased risk of heart disease, breast and uterine cancer, diabetes, high blood pressure, and stroke. The good news is that I can help you lose pounds and maintain the ideal weight for your body in a healthy way, without unbalanced diets or other gimmicks.

After age 20, a woman's metabolism slows down by 10 percent every decade. So, it is logical that, by age 40, you need to cut down on your quantity of food and number of calories to keep the same weight that you had in your 20s. This is difficult to do for many women, and it is tempting to look for a quick fix, but fad diets come with a high price: The yo-yo effect of big swings in weight can stress your internal organs and even result in degenerative diseases. Relying on weight-loss pills without adopting appropriate nutritional and lifestyle regimens can cause side effects such as nervousness, insomnia, high blood pressure, menstrual disruption, hair loss, heart attack, and stroke.

The Chinese Weight-Management Philosophy

Two out of three people in the United States are overweight, and Americans spend vast sums on weight-loss programs, with dismal results. The failure to contain the nation's waist size reveals a fundamental flaw in the approach to the problem. Effective, sustained, healthy weight management must take into account physical and emotional causes and address each person's underlying issues.

40

In the long history of Chinese medicine, we have observed that each person is born with an elemental constitutional type that manifests certain physical and emotional attributes. Eating foods that benefit and correspond to your particular type in the Five Elements archetype helps to maximize health and balance in your body, mind, and spirit. In this chapter, you will learn how to determine your elemental constitutional type in the Chinese medical model and eat accordingly. I will show you how to use moderate cardiovascular exercise for circulation, mind-body meditation to reduce stress, massage and acupuncture to stoke the metabolic fire, and Chinese herbal supplements to rid the body of dampness, mucus, and toxins.

Imbalance in the function of the thyroid, pancreas, ovaries, and adrenal glands can contribute to weight gain as women get older. In Western medicine the metabolic slowdown is often attributed to waning activity of the thyroid, which regulates metabolism. But this in turn may be due to emotional stresses that weaken the adrenal gland—the seat of your survival abilities—triggering a cascade of metabolic reactions that affect everything from blood sugar to fat storage. Our bodies' stress mechanisms evolved in an era when humans were both hunters and hunted; today, they react to the constant pressures of modern life and work by producing stress hormones, keeping your body perpetually overstimulated. Adrenal overstimulation causes the body to conserve energy and pack on fat as it would have to survive days of privation while hiding from predators. You can tell your body that you are not actually in survival mode by eating frequent small meals and using meditation to relax.

Two Possible Factors: Estrogen Dominance and Insulin Resistance

Aging in women corresponds with a decline in estrogen, but many women actually find themselves in estrogen dominance—the condition of having too much estrogen—in perimenopause. The decline in hormone production by the ovaries and uterus, coupled with a diet of refined carbohydrates, can cause the adrenal glands, fat cells, kidneys, and liver to compensate by producing more of the hormone, often pushing the body's estrogen to excessive levels. Environmental toxins like PCBs and phthalates in plastics, formaldehyde in carpets and furniture, and paraben preservatives in personal care products are all *xenoestrogens* (substances that mimic estrogen), which enter the body and contribute to further imbalance. This overload is associated with increased risk of cancer, diabetes, obesity, edema, cystic breasts and ovaries, endometriosis, uterine fibroids, and high blood pressure. This chapter shows you how to rid your body of toxins through simple cleansing techniques and to restore hormonal balance through mind-body exercise that will help you reach a healthy weight.

Good digestion and proper pancreas function are essential to maintaining optimum metabolism. Together, the spleen, stomach, and pancreas break down food, separate essential nutrients from waste, and transport the fuel to the cells. When digestive function is disrupted, bloating, gas, weight gain, fatigue, constipation or diarrhea, abdominal pain, and menstrual disorders ensue. Moreover, when the pancreas releases too much insulin due to *insulin resistance*—a condition in which cells are unable to take in glucose—this forces the conversion of glucose to stored fat. Water retention, high cholesterol, acne, cysts in breasts and ovaries, hair loss, and excess facial hair can also result, a condition known as *Syndrome X*. Healthy food, regular exercise, and stress reduction are key to overcoming and preventing insulin resistance.

The Mind and Digestion

Emotional symptoms associated with digestive imbalance in Chinese medical science include melancholy, obsessive thoughts, worry, restless sleep, and poor concentration. Often, digestive problems are at the root of these emotional symptoms. Stressful emotions, in turn, take a toll on the digestive system, causing a wide range of abnormalities. Interestingly, studies have now confirmed the existence of an independent network of more than 100 billion neurons in the gut, where 95 percent of the neurotransmitter *serotonin* (a calming hormone) is found. This finding has led some to call the gut our "second brain." To achieve your ideal weight, it is essential for you to practice effective stress management behaviors and strategies. I will teach you some of these practices here.

For the modern woman, the pressures of daily life may include primary responsibility for child-rearing in addition to serving as the sole or partial breadwinner for the family. She rarely has time or resources to enjoy herself, which leads her to seek comfort in food. And food does the job, albeit temporarily, but it also jumpstarts an addictive cycle. Most women choose comfort foods like chocolate, candies, soda, and simple starches such as refined pastries, fries, and chips—the very foods that cause blood sugar imbalance and weight gain. To overcome emotional eating, you need to change the role of food in your life from feel-good crutch to nourishing sustenance. We try to help our female patients to develop emotional fulfillment elsewhere in life—from improving intimacy in their personal relationships to engaging in creative endeavors, travel, or community volunteerism—rather than drugging themselves with food.

With the simple principles and easy-to-implement methods outlined in this book, you can use your inherent mind-body connection to begin losing weight naturally and sustainably, while improving your health and energy.

Diet for the
Second Spring

When women undergo menopause, the need for certain
nutrients increases. You'll require more amino acids, and
protein plays a more important role than before. What
should you eat to stay healthy and keep from gaining
weight? The formula is simple. Animal protein should
make up 25 percent of your diet: seafood, egg (or just the
egg white, if you are concerned about cholesterol), chicken,
turkey, and lamb. Eat three 4-ounce portions—the size
of a deck of cards—per day. Fruits and vegetables should
account for a full 50 percent of your diet, for their bounteous
benefits in antioxidants, vitamins, and fiber. The final 25
percent should be divided among raw nuts and seeds,
rich in fatty acids; beans and legumes, which are natural
sources of estrogens; and whole grains, which help
regulate blood sugar levels. Cut back on carbohydrates
such as sugar, white flour, and alcohol.

Spread your meals,
not your waistline

After age 20, your metabolism slows down by about 10 percent every decade. This may explain why you can't eat the same quantity of food you did when you were younger. Even when your level of activity and exercise remains the same, eating the same amount of food may make you gain weight. But you can reverse this metabolic decline by changing your eating habits. A pattern of five small meals a day instead of three larger ones keeps the metabolism going without storing up extra reserves. It is never a good idea to eat big meals because your body can only use a certain amount of food, depending on your activities, and will stockpile the rest as fat. Ideally, you'll eat breakfast, a snack, lunch, a snack, and dinner—small amounts and, of course, all healthy food. By eating small meals, you keep the fire burning and won't put anything in storage.

Fennel for
Digestive Health

An often unacknowledged change during perimenopause and menopause is a decline in digestive health. The secretion of gastric juices decreases with age, resulting in abdominal pain, bloating, and gas. Chinese medicine also recognizes that an emotional element can come into play because the liver is highly sensitive to mood and feelings, and a weak flow of liver energy may manifest as bloating or flatulence. A common remedy in China is fennel, the plant with delicious, fragrant leaves eaten raw in salads; fennel seed is often used as a spice in dishes with meat, beans, or legumes. Fennel helps digestion in two ways: It stimulates the production of gastric juices and also soothes the nervous system, regulating the action of the muscles that line the intestine. Use it regularly in cooking, with extra portions when you are experiencing gastric distress.

Don't douse that
fire in your belly

Ancient medical traditions, including those of Hippocrates, Maimonides, and the Yellow Emperor, have universally recognized that different foods have warming or cooling properties in the body. When you eat raw food, its energetic property is *cold*. For someone with a *hot* condition or body type—typically quick-tempered, thirsty, excessively hungry, and constipated—cold or *cooling* foods like raw vegetables are the appropriate counterbalance. When my patients with *cold* conditions or body types eat too much raw and cold-temperature food, however, they react with abdominal bloating, gas, diarrhea, and lethargy. Cooking partially breaks down your food, making the nutrients accessible to your body's systems; for example, more *lycopene*, an essential carotenoid antioxidant that has been found to reduce the risks of heart disease, macular degeneration, as well as prostate and other cancers, is more available in cooked tomatoes than in uncooked. Eating raw food all the time requires more energy for digestion and tends to put out the digestive fire, leaving you colder and more tired. A little raw food is fine, but eat mostly cooked dishes to keep those belly fires burning.

Can you eat meat and lose fat?

Conjugated linoleic acid (CLA) is a natural fatty acid found in beef and lamb, especially the grass-fed kind, and also in eggs. This powerful antioxidant has a wealth of benefits: It supports healthy immune response to joint inflammation, maintains healthy blood glucose and insulin, and, in animal studies, hindered the growth of tumors in breast, skin, and colon tissues. But CLA is best known for its ability to improve the ratio of fat-to-lean body mass. So if you want to reduce body fat but don't want to give up your red meat, go ahead and eat it—just be sure to consume only free-range, grass-fed, and hormone- and antibiotic-free lean meat, and eat it no more than three times a week. You also should exercise every day to get the full benefits of CLA. You can also take it in supplement form, usually 3 to 4 grams per day.

Food and drink...
don't mix!

If you are lavishing your body with the finest nutrition, that's wonderful. Now you need to ensure that your system can make use of the food you eat. Drink your fluids in between meals so that you do not dilute your gastric juices at mealtime. Consuming beverages during a meal weakens the teamwork of the spleen and stomach, and interferes with the organs' function of proper digestion and absorption of nutrients. Wait at least 30 minutes after eating before you drink fluids. In between meals, sip herbal teas, water, and vegetable juices; avoid coffee, sodas, and other sugary beverages. Similarly, fruits with high water content should be eaten between meals, especially melons of all kinds. Soups are the exception to the rule: A broth of nutritious ingredients is actually easier to assimilate.

Three ways to stay trim and ward off diabetes

When your body lacks insulin, or can't use it, you're going to get fat. The cells in the pancreas that produce insulin decline in function by an average of 10 to 20 percent by age 30, and women's tendency to develop *insulin resistance* (cellular inability to utilize insulin in the blood) increases dramatically around menopause. This can lead to type 2 diabetes, which is eight times more common in people 60 and older than in those under 40. Three ways to help reverse insulin resistance:

1) Take cinnamon, as a spice or as tea, to control blood sugar. I suggest that my patients take 1 to 2 grams in food or two to three cups of cinnamon tea daily.

2) Use acupressure. Locate the point four finger-widths beneath the indentation of your outer knee. This spot (Stomach-36) regulates metabolism and can increase your cells' sensitivity to insulin. Press it for one minute, then release. Repeat three times. Do this twice a day for two to four weeks.

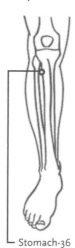

Stomach-36

3) Perform cardio exercise. Just 30 to 40 minutes daily will boost your cells' ability to take up sugar from the bloodstream.

Watercress fights
water weight

Watercress, a piquant green you can use to spice up a salad, contains a rich supply of vitamins A and E as well as the minerals calcium, magnesium, potassium, manganese, phosphorous, iodine, and zinc. According to Chinese medicine, watercress clears heat and lubricates the lungs, so it is an excellent remedy for cough, sore throat, and upper respiratory inflammation. Most significantly for older women, it is also a natural diuretic that helps alleviate the bloated sensation and excess water retention that can occur during menopause. The cooling properties of watercress also calm restlessness, so toss some into your salad on hot summer days when nothing seems to satisfy.

NAC off toxins and pounds

Amino acids play many important roles in maintaining your health and restoring it when you get ill. One in particular, N-acetyl cysteine (NAC), is a major component of hair *and* a strong antioxidant that bolsters your immune system. It helps to detoxify a damaging substance called *acetaldehyde*, which enters your system when you are exposed to cigarette smoke, car exhaust, nail polish remover, and certain other pollutants; it is also produced in your body when you drink alcohol or have a yeast infection. NAC even acts to remove mercury, a highly toxic heavy metal, and to protect tissues from free radicals associated with UV radiation and muscular exertion. It has recently been discovered by bodybuilders because it helps to build muscle and promotes the burning of fat. Typical dose is 600 mg per day.

Magnolia eases
nervous eating

Chronic stress seems to be our national disease. Millions experience one or more of its symptoms: nervous tension, restless sleep, difficulty focusing, irritability, and, especially, eating disorders. People often respond to situational stress by eating comfort foods like ice cream, cookies, and chocolate. When the stress becomes chronic, over-eating becomes the norm. To break the pattern, natural Chinese medicine comes to the rescue with the versatile magnolia, used to encourage weight loss and to counter allergic reactions. The bark regulates appetite, improves digestion, and reduces swelling and bloating; the flower is an effective remedy for allergies and sinus conditions. Studies show that magnolia contains a phytochemical called honokiol with antistress properties that prove useful in appetite control and weight management. Consider taking a magnolia supplement by itself or in formulations with other herbs, in tea or capsules available at health food stores, online, and from acupuncturists and Chinese herbalists.

Eat melon,
don't look like one!

If you want to lose weight, you're probably thinking of how you can eat less, but here's a traditional remedy that involves something you add to your diet. Bitter melon, also known as balsam pear, is a traditional remedy for being overweight, diabetes, and various infections. Its cleansing and mildly laxative properties flush the system of toxins and promote natural weight loss. The melon contains vitamins A, B1, B3, and C as well as numerous phytonutrients—including antioxidants like lutein, lycopene, and zeaxanthin—plus twice the beta-carotene of broccoli, twice the calcium of spinach, and twice the potassium of bananas! A good source of dietary fiber, bitter melon is widely sold in Asian markets. Typically, it is stuffed like zucchini: Discard the seeds inside and fill with ground poultry or red meat to buffer its bitter taste quality. You get used to its unusual taste, as you do to eating bitter greens.

Eating out
the smart way

The standard dinner at a restaurant begins with an appetizer, followed by salad, an entrée, dessert, and coffee. We often down all this with wine or cocktails. It is amazing to me that we don't get heartburn more often. To avoid overeating when you eat out, follow these simple strategies:

Stick with appetizers. In the United States, the entrées on a menu are almost always too big for one person. Try ordering appetizers instead. A couple of these small dishes should fill you up and give you some variety.

Ask for a box. When you order an entrée, especially pasta, ask for a box when the entrée arrives and box up half of it before you start eating—or ask the waiter to do this before the food is brought to you. That way you won't try to finish the whole plate.

Split your order. If you are eating with a spouse or a close friend or relative, offer to split the entrée order with him or her. Each of you can pick an appetizer for yourselves in addition. You'll save money and your waistline at the same time.

Refuse the dessert menu. When the waiter asks if you want the dessert menu, politely refuse. Or order an herbal tea such as chamomile, peppermint, or orange spice, which will help your digestion, and add a spoonful of honey.

No time for exercise?
Think physical

A formalized exercise program is ideal for losing weight, but it is not the only way. If you feel overwhelmed by the idea of fitting a new routine into your schedule, instead of thinking "exercise," think "physical activity." If you have a sedentary job requiring you to sit for long hours during the day, you can use your break periods and the time before and after work to invigorate yourself. Before you grab a cup of coffee or sit down to lunch, walk up a few flights of stairs. Park a few blocks away from work, or better yet, walk or bike to and from the office. Try to engage in more physical exertion on weekends, such as mowing the lawn with a manual mower, gardening, vacuuming, and washing the car. Participate in a community walkathon; volunteer to clean up parkland; coach your kid's soccer team— whatever gets you outdoors and moving.

Watch for
hidden sugar

Ever pick up a sugar-free energy or granola bar only
to take a bite and find it sweeter than traditional candy?
It says it is sweetened by fruit juice only, but a closer look
at the label reveals that it is concentrated fruit juice—which
contains more calories than sugar would. Don't be fooled:
When it comes to weight management, calories are
calories. A simple carbohydrate, sugar belongs to one
of our necessary food groups. There is nothing wrong with
it unless you consume too much. If you have a sweet tooth,
instead of turning to artificial sweeteners, try naturally
low- or no-calorie substances from nature. The natural
herb stevia and erythritol, a sugar alcohol from fermented
fruits, both contain no calories. Luo han guo, a Chinese
herb traditionally used for cough and sore throat, is now
available as an extract combined with the vegetable fiber
inulin; the mixture, Sweet Fiber, serves as a no-calorie
natural sweetener with the added benefit of fiber.

Seek your best weight— not someone else's

You are a unique individual, and your ideal proportions are yours alone. Don't expect to become someone you're not, like a fashion model. It won't work, and then you may eat more to allay your anxiety—a setup for failure. Take these tips.

Focus on fitness, not weight. Fit means feeling great and being able to move unhampered by your physical condition. It also means fitting comfortably in a chair, an airplane seat, and your car. Work on getting healthy and fit, and in the process you will lose weight. Focusing only on your weight creates unnecessary stress.

Resize your expectations to match your genetics. Your ideal weight depends to some extent on your family history. For example, if you have a genetic history of heart disease, diabetes, and stroke, an apple shape is not healthy for you. Reducing your waist and bust size will reduce your risk of these diseases. Conversely, if osteoporosis runs in your family, you may want to carry a little extra weight to keep more calcium in your bones.

Allow for some fat in the right places. Fat is not always the enemy. It helps protect bones from injury during a fall, and the fat layer under the skin lessens wrinkles and softens an overly angular face. Fat cells are also your source of estrogen after menopause. It's better to be a plum than a prune, so keep a little fat where it does some good!

Choose the right fats

In some countries, lard and butter are the standard cooking oils. No wonder heart disease is consistently the number-one killer in the world. Animal fats are saturated fats, which contribute to bad cholesterol, weight gain, and plaque buildup in our delicate circulatory system. Mono-unsaturated and polyunsaturated fats like vegetable, nut, and seed oils, on the other hand, increase good cholesterol and protect you from heart disease, inflammation, and premature skin aging. These include olive oil, rice bran oil, walnut oil, flaxseed oil, peanut oil, and sesame oil. The worst offenders of all are trans fats. These are not natural fats but are manufactured by partially hydrogenating plant oils to give them a longer shelf life. Margarine and shortening are two examples widely used in fast-food restaurants and packaged snacks. Your body has a hard time processing trans fats, which increase bad cholesterol and your risk of diabetes and stroke. Some studies directly implicate trans fats in producing the unattractive rippling fatty deposits known as *cellulite*.

Watch that
bread and pasta

Food staples around the world tend to be refined bread, pasta, rice, and corn, carbohydrates that have been found to be the culprits in serious conditions like diabetes, stroke, and heart disease as well as arthritis, attention deficit disorder, and allergies. There is no question that refined carbohydrates contribute directly to weight gain. So change to whole grains to get complex carbohydrates—whole wheat bread, brown rice, whole grain pasta—and try diversifying beyond the typical. For example, quinoa and amaranth are two tasty grains rich in protein and easy to cook. Millet, sorghum, and buckwheat are packed with B vitamins and add variety to your diet. While whole grains are very nutritious and provide fiber, an important part of our diet, eat them moderately for optimum help with your weight management goals. Eating less of your daily grain intake during the day and more of it in the evening can also help your energy and sleep cycles.

The Chinese elements:
Find your type
for ideal weight

In Chinese medicine, each person is considered to have an elemental constitutional type. The five different types—wood, fire, earth, metal, and water—have different gifts and vulnerabilities. Certain foods that are healthy for one type must be avoided by another. No one diet is right for everyone. The complex interactions of your metabolism, emotions, mind, spirit, genetics, and other factors cannot be addressed in full here, but chances are you will recognize yourself, in whole or in large part, among the constitutions discussed below. Peruse the lists of recommended foods for your type and foods to avoid. If you eat according to the needs of your constitutional element, you can arrive at your ideal weight—and the state of well-being you deserve.

Wood element: intense personality, headache prone

People whose elemental type is Wood usually have a facial structure that is rectangular and muscular, with an olive complexion. They tend to be highly motivated and have a very strong personality. Often identified as Type A sorts, they may be high energy, confident, intense, smart, decisive, responsible, and authoritative. Wood types tend to command respect but are also prone to stubbornness and are sometimes overbearing and controlling. They are susceptible to disorders of the liver, nervous system—especially the brain—throat, bronchial tubes, esophagus, and stomach. They tend to suffer from frequent headaches, eye disorders, nerve pain, neck and shoulder pain, throat constriction, acid reflux disorder, and high blood pressure.

This is the health picture of someone who is over-stressed, as those with Wood constitutions often are. They can benefit from practicing meditation and yoga on a regular basis. Competitive sports are not ideal recreation activities for Wood types, who are already too goal-oriented. Instead, they should engage in hiking, sailing, birdwatching—anything that is an end in itself.

RECOMMENDED: Beet (and greens), burdock root, carrot (and greens), collard greens, Swiss chard, kale, mustard greens, parsley, dulse, Irish moss, dandelion, spinach, turnip, yam, sweet potato, tomato, asparagus, corn, pearl barley, barley, brussels sprouts, broccoli, rhubarb, squash, winter melon (and its seed), zucchini, pumpkin (and seed), flaxseed (and oil), psyllium seed, sunflower seed, olive (and oil), honey, seaweed, mushrooms (shiitake, porcini, portobello), bamboo shoots, peppermint, spearmint, lentil, split pea, artichoke, mung bean, soybean (including tofu and miso), black bean, grape, loquat, kiwi, nectarine, litchi fruit, plum, raspberry, blueberry, cranberry, strawberry, basil, sesame seed (and oil), rice vinegar, sage, bran, chicken, turkey, fish, egg whites.

AVOID: Deep-fried and fatty foods, alcohol, caffeine, sugar, overly sour foods, iced drinks, dairy products, wheat, barley, yeast, pork, red meat, peanut, banana, fruit juice, orange, artificial sweetener.

Fire element: quick mind, heart problems

This constitutional type tends to be very passionate, excitable, sensitive, and impatient. She has a triangular face that narrows at the chin, with prominent features and a slightly reddish complexion. A Fire person is very much a quick study, has an eye for details, and is ambitious and persistent but frustrates quickly and does not easily adapt to change. Sociable and articulate as a rule, they may nonetheless have a hard time getting along with others due to their strong egos, and may thus become isolated. Fire element types are susceptible to circulatory and cardiovascular problems such as hypertension and heart conditions, varicose and spider veins, as well as anxiety, insomnia, palpitations, stress, neck and shoulder tightness and soreness, toothache, constipation, and menstrual problems.

If you are a Fire type it is very important to schedule your time, especially during the midlife transition, and make sure to set some aside for yourself. This means not just being alone, but thinking seriously about your own well-being. Start a journal if you haven't already. What brings you joy? Remind yourself that you deserve it and make a place for it in your life.

RECOMMENDED: Bok choy, red cabbage, red chard, turnip, radish, celery, spinach, red potato, red bell pepper, cauliflower, carrot, mustard greens, tomato, mushroom, buckwheat, beet root (and greens), celery, asparagus, lemon, sunflower seed, pear, pomegranate, mulberry, red apple, wheat bran, raspberry, boysenberry, strawberry, cranberry, brown rice, quinoa, amaranth, adzuki bean, kidney bean, soybean, tofu, red jujube date, coconut, carob, hawthorn berry, rosemary, tarragon, savory, safflower, endive, chili pepper, chicken, shrimp, fish, goat dairy, egg, olive oil, flaxseed oil, canola oil.

AVOID: Rich and greasy foods, cow dairy, deep-fried and fatty foods, red meat, refined sugar, sweets, alcohol, caffeine, wheat, yeast, overly spicy foods, artificial sweetener.

Earth element: giving and nurturing, suffers stomach ailments

Sincere, easygoing, giving and nurturing, the Earth elemental type tends to make friends easily. She takes a conservative, methodical approach and is generally not the initiator. Earth types tend to have oval faces that are full, fleshy, and slightly yellow in complexion. They are imaginative but prone to overthinking and worry. They usually have big appetites and may overindulge. Earth element people tend to have digestive and intestinal problems including disorders of pancreas, stomach, spleen, and intestines; they may suffer from ulcers, inflammation of the intestines, diarrhea, constipation, bloating, water retention, muscular weakness, and low energy.

If your element is Earth, you feel most content when you are in the company of other people. You thrive on their energy and you nurture them in return. When you are out of balance you may become needy—wanting more and more affection—or give too much of yourself, becoming a pushover. Now is the time to work on your self-reliance and to develop the skill of setting boundaries in your life.

RECOMMENDED: Alfalfa sprouts, carrot, cauliflower, celery, daikon radish, mushroom, potato, seaweed, snow pea, spinach, yam, sweet potato, hawthorn berry, guava, persimmon, kumquat, strawberry, papaya, blueberry, pearl barley, tofu, bamboo shoot, bok choy, cilantro, lotus root, pumpkin, all squash, soybean (and sprouts), golden apple, grapefruit, lemon, lime, eggs, turnip, prune, fig, barley, rice, buckwheat, millet, oat, yellow bell pepper, green bean, kale, lotus seed, mustard green, parsley, red grape, cherry, jujube date, mango, pineapple, plum, garbanzo bean, adzuki bean, lima bean, pea, beef, fish, lamb, anise, basil, fennel, dill, cayenne, cumin, ginger, brown rice vinegar, mustard seed.

AVOID: Iced drinks, raw vegetables and fruits, dairy, alcohol, caffeine, refined sugar, deep-fried and fatty foods, process and refined foods, wheat, yeast, pork, melon, artificial sweetener.

Metal element: intellectual and organized, frequent colds and flu

The classic facial structure for people of the metal type is round and wide, with a prominent nose and fair complexion. Metal types tend to be very intellectual, articulate, rational, meticulous, and organized. When they focus their energy on a single task, they are persistent and usually follow through to the end. Yet their overly optimistic outlook, curious nature, and ability to see myriad possibilities can lead to excessive deliberating. This causes Metal constitutional types to change their minds too often and spread themselves too thin, thereby becoming scattered and unfocused. Because they are so good at what they do, they tend to become overextended. Metal types tend to suffer respiratory conditions such as sinusitis, allergies, and asthma and often fall prey to laryngitis, colitis, upper back pain, colds and flu, and diseases affecting the mouth, teeth, skin, and bone marrow.

It's especially important for Metal types to establish regular mealtimes rather than eating erratically. However, do encourage spontaneity in your creative life, to counteract your hyperrational side. Aerobic exercise will benefit your health—and stop smoking now!

RECOMMENDED: Burdock root, cabbage, carrot, daikon radish (and seed), seaweed, agar, spinach, watercress, apple, banana, prune, fig, mulberry, peach, Asian pear, Bartlett pear, persimmon, strawberry, soybean, tofu, asparagus, bok choy, beet, cauliflower, egg whites, eggplant, white potato, pumpkin (and seed), snow pea, jicama, barley, brown or wild rice, millet, mushroom, winter melon seed, turnip, cantaloupe, apricot, parsnip, scallion, onion, pine nut, walnut, ginger, horseradish, mustard greens, molasses, rice vinegar, garlic, berries, pineapple, sesame seed, fennel, okra, papaya, jujube date, cherry, peanut, pea, olive, almond, white bean, thyme, string bean, fish, chicken, turkey.

AVOID: All dairy products, alcohol, overly spicy foods, iced drinks, caffeine, refined sugar, deep-fried and fatty foods, wheat, barbecued foods, red meat, dried or dehydrated products, artificial sweetener.

Water element: strong willpower, hormone problems

If a person's element is Water, she will likely have strong willpower and endurance, yet can also seem timid, hesitant, unsure of herself. Perhaps she is physically weak. With this duality, people with Water constitutions may become too dependent on others or go to extremes in decision-making, alienating those around them. They are usually deep thinkers, content with the pleasures of the mind. Water types typically have square, filled-out face, large ears, and a dark complexion. They may age prematurely and are susceptible to urinary, genital, and reproductive ailments such as infertility and impotence; their health problems tend to involve the kidneys, bladder, urinary tract, ovaries, hormonal system, and lower back.

Are you a Water element? Drink lots of water! It's not as simplistic as it sounds: Fluids clear out the kidneys, which are your weak point. It's also important for you to nurture your social relations and not spend too much time alone. You may be very self-sufficient, but this can become coldness and detachment from others when you are out of balance.

RECOMMENDED: Broccoli, carrot, celery, blue corn, cucumber, daikon radish, eggplant, lotus root, seaweed, snow pea, soybean (and sprouts), avocado, spinach, zucchini, watercress, watermelon (and seed), mulberry, pear, millet, pearl barley, amaranth, quinoa, black bean, bamboo shoot, blueberry, blackberry, cabbage, leek, shiitake mushroom, potato, squash, winter melon, cantaloupe, chives, shallot, jujube date, green bean, mustard greens, parsnip, grape, raspberry, black bean, cashew, chestnut, walnut, sesame seed, venison, livers, chicken, beef, lamb, fish, adzuki bean, peanut, pea, lotus seed, green bean, coconut, black rice, wild rice, oregano.

AVOID: Overly salty foods, alcohol, caffeine, fatty and deep-fried foods, iced drinks, raw vegetables and fruits, dairy, refined sugar, deep-fried and fatty foods, wheat, yeast, artificial sweetener.

CHAPTER 3

Create Higher Energy

IN CHINESE MEDICINE, energy equals quality of life. We use the word *qi* (pronounced "chee") to refer to the life force, the energy that allows you to live your life passionately and vigorously. One of the hallmarks of aging is a decline in qi, which can be very noticeable in women in menopause. Of all the changes happening in the body at midlife, waning energy is perhaps the most common complaint from my female patients. Many women come to me feeling tired and listless, saying that things they used to do easily now seem to take more effort. Well, there are good reasons. Biology dictates that in menopause and thereafter a woman's body not only shuts down its reproductive processes but also switches from expansion mode to conservation mode. This process can begin as early as 35. Many women have more demands—kids AND elderly parent care AND a job—creating less and less energy as life goes on. This can force an adjustment in your activity level if you do not address your energy loss. Conditions like diabetes, obesity, and poor circulation only compound the problem.

Energy is something we take for granted until we don't have it. In our fast-paced society, most people are on the run from the moment they wake until they collapse into bed at night. They keep going until they run out of steam. Most people's energy decline doesn't happen overnight but sneaks up on them over time, until gradually they need more and more stimulants to carry out their normal routines. For others, the loss of energy has a sudden, dramatic onset, whether from a lingering illness, acute depression from emotional trauma, or adrenal burnout from prolonged stress. It is important to remember to take care of your adrenal glands, the seat of your survival mechanism, by dealing with the stress in your life in healthy ways—particularly by using brief meditations to relax. You want to avoid activating them too often, because adrenal exhaustion can lead to a serious health breakdown.

When Your Body Attacks Itself

Your immune function has a direct effect on your energy level. When the immune system is busy fighting an infection, it is using all your body's resources to defend against the invaders, and you typically feel very low in energy. Likewise, if your immune system is busy fighting enemies from within, such as toxins, allergens, or other foreign particles carried in the body, it can produce an autoimmune response in the form of inflammation. In other words, your body thinks your own cells are the enemy, and your health suffers collateral damage that can include eczema, arthritis, and lupus, to name a few possible outcomes. Autoimmunity occurs more frequently as women approach menopause due to shifts in hormonal output that upset the balance of the immune system. Besides inflammation, the most common symptom of autoimmune disorder is fatigue. Balancing your immune system is key to restoring vitality.

The Life Force: Your Inheritance and Your Responsibility

In Chinese medical science, declining energy during your transition through menopause is attributed to depletion of both prenatal and postnatal qi. Prenatal qi is what you inherit from your parents: your genetic potential and tendencies. Postnatal qi is energy from the nourishment your body receives after you are born. This means both what you eat and how well your digestive system transforms your food into the critical nutrients that fuel your cells.

Optimal digestion is essential for abundant energy. The digestive function is carried out by many organs in close cooperation, mainly the stomach, spleen, pancreas, small intestine, and liver. In Chinese medicine, this collective function is called the *spleen organ network*, and it governs not only digestion but also the muscles, blood vessels, thinking process, blood production, and qi—your cells' vital energy. When the network breaks down or is weakened, anemia, broken capillaries, muscle weakness, cognitive decline, low energy, and indigestion may ensue. Later in this chapter I share with you the natural herbs, supplements, and diet tips that can help strengthen your spleen network and boost your qi.

Poor diet begets poor energy. Under normal circumstances your body actually prefers to derive its energy from fat. The hunter-gatherer lifestyle of our ancestors meant that food supply was inconsistent. A good catch might be followed by days or weeks of a subsistence diet. To survive, the human body developed efficient ways of storing energy as fat and converting the fat back into energy. A balanced diet of proteins from vegetable or animal sources, fats from meats and nuts, and complex carbohydrates from vegetables and fruits is extremely important in your energy equation. Refined carbohydrates, on the other hand, such as white bread, pasta, pastries, white rice, and cereals are modern inventions that are unfamiliar to your body and wreak havoc on your energy-production chain.

Oxygen Fuels Your Cells

While your spleen network extracts nutrition from your food, the nutrient synthesis must mix with oxygen to produce useful qi. The oxygen from the air we breathe is carried by hemoglobin in the blood to every cell in the body. Oxygen, fats, and carbohydrates arrive at your cells to be processed into fuel by little organelles within the cells called *mitochondria*. This is called *aerobic energy production*, the best and most efficient kind. The two best ways to ensure adequate oxygen intake are to practice breathing meditations and to exercise every day. Abdominal breathing, the standard technique in most meditation practices, not only boosts oxygen absorption, it also helps to detoxify the body. Exercise also increases oxygen but, when overdone, causes a buildup of toxic gases and lactic acid, which does more harm than good. For an ideal combination of moderate exercise and meditative breathing, I practice qi gong or tai chi, which have been shown in studies to elevate the oxygen saturation of your cells.

Many women find themselves low in aerobic energy function, so their bodies instead rely on anaerobic energy production—the manufacture of short bursts of energy for emergency purposes. This generates waste products like free radicals and lactic acid, which accelerate aging and exhaust the adrenal glands. When toxins such as heavy metals, pesticides, and dioxins accumulate in the body, the mitochondria cannot work properly, forcing your body to switch to anaerobic energy production. In recent studies, researchers have focused on mitochondria breakdown as the cause of aging. In this chapter, I will recommend certain nutrients that are beneficial for mitochondrial function and show you how to shift your body back to aerobic energy production.

Menopause does not have to be the start of a downhill slide in your energy and vitality. Using proper herbs, super foods, acupressure, exercise, and dietary supplements, you can tap into the energy within your being and maintain your equilibrium and health.

Bite-size changes
to ease into health

Trying to alter your habits and routines can be daunting, even when you know the changes are for the better. Here's a modest program that will help you get on track without feeling overwhelmed:

Week 1—Drink a lot more water this week. In between meals, drink 40 ounces of water a day (5 8-ounce glasses). And use up or clean out all the food that is currently in your kitchen to make way for new healthier food.

Week 2—Eat five to seven colorful fruits and vegetables every day.

Week 3—Carry dried fruits and nuts with you as healthy snacks to replace any unhealthy ones you usually eat. Eat hummus instead of butter on your bagel.

Week 4—Replace all the white food in your pantry with brown food. Go to your health food store and bring back brown rice instead of white, whole wheat bread instead of white bread, buckwheat pasta instead of white, and so on.

You're already on your way to a healthier you!

Green is good for your blood

The green pigment in plants, *chlorophyll*, is structurally similar to the hemoglobin in the human body—the iron-containing element in blood. Women at midlife are vulnerable to anemia, and plant chlorophyll is the perfect tonic. It increases red blood cell production and improves oxygenation, detoxification, and circulation. Be sure to eat several servings of fresh green vegetables every day. In supplement form, take advantage of the rich sources of chlorophyll found in barley, wheat grass, alfalfa, and sea-weed such as blue-green algae, spirulina, and chlorella. Mix a powder of any of the above into water, juice, or green tea for a fortifying, purifying tonic for the blood.

Eat late,
wake up tired

In our hectic modern life, many people don't get out of work until late, and that usually means eating a late dinner. Whether it's due to work, household tasks, or some other cause, eating late spells trouble for your health on many fronts. First of all, your body will be digesting your dinner while you are trying to sleep, so you won't feel rested in the morning. Many people who eat late wake up tired and foggy-headed. In addition, the liver works on detoxification while you sleep at night and can't do its job right when there is food to digest as well. So when you eat late, you overburden your body, stress out your liver, and interfere with a good night's sleep—that's a big price to pay for a couple of extra hours at the office.

Magnesium
fights fatigue

Every time your body produces energy, your cells' *mitochrondria*—their tiny power generators—require magnesium. It's an essential mineral, but many people don't get enough of it, because two common dietary habits leach magnesium from our bodies: too much salt and too much dairy. Moreover, due to the popularity of overprocessed foods, most of us simply don't get enough magnesium in the first place. For example, rice bran contains a rich supply of the mineral, but bran is found only in brown rice—white rice has none. Likewise, there is plenty of magnesium in wheat germ, but it's eliminated in white bread and white pasta. Now you see why eating whole grains is so important! Seeds such as pumpkin, sesame, and sunflower seeds are full of magnesium; so are nuts, especially almonds, Brazil nuts, and cashews. Magnesium also benefits heart function, relieves muscle cramps, softens stools, and protects skin from UV damage. In capsule form, the suggested dosage is 500 mg of magnesium daily.

Probiotics keep digestion on track

Our bodies host plenty of guests in the form of beneficial, healthy bacteria that live inside us. At one time or another, most people have used antibiotics, reinforcements that Western doctors prescribe to help us fight off harmful infections. Unfortunately, these drugs also wipe out the helpful organisms that play an important role in our digestive process. When this happens, you want to replenish the intestinal flora with probiotics. There are several types, and fortunately you can obtain most through natural food. For a rich, readily available source of lactobacillus, eat yogurt, preferably goat yogurt, easier to digest than the kind made from cow's milk. Additional sources include sauerkraut, miso, tempeh, and soybeans. Immediately after a course of antibiotics you may wish to recharge your system with probiotic supplements, which are found with refrigerated items in health food stores. Be sure they contain bifidobacteria, enterococci, and saccharomyces as well as lactobacillus. Always take them on an empty stomach.

The joy
of sax

Lung capacity is directly proportional to vitality and longevity. If the lungs aren't working optimally to supply the body with oxygen, all the metabolic processes go haywire and you are at increased risk of heart disease, deteriorating mental function, nerve damage, cancer, vision loss, and countless other health problems. By midlife, many people have compromised the health of their lungs by smoking or simply by breathing urban air with its payload of particulates and other toxic pollutants. What to do? How about making music to improve your health! Try playing a wind instrument—saxophone, flute, trumpet, trombone, clarinet, even a pennywhistle. If you've never done it before, take lessons and get the dual benefit of exercising the lungs and stimulating the brain with something new. Practicing for as little as 10 or 15 minutes per day will expand your lung capacity.

Discover the
ideal antioxidant

To be sure you're getting the full effect of vitamins C and E as antioxidants, help them with alpha-lipoic acid, another high-powered antioxidant with an unusual characteristic: It fights free radicals in the watery parts of your cells, just as vitamin C does, and also in the fatty parts, where vitamin E operates. When these two vitamins would otherwise be exhausted, alpha-lipoic acid renews their activity, turning the by-products of metabolism into new antioxidant compounds. The acid is an important nutrient for converting food into cellular energy and prevents nerve damage from age-related ailments such as diabetes, Parkinson's, and Alzheimer's disease. This "ideal antioxidant," as some researchers call it, helps your body get the most energy out of what you eat as well as your vitamin supplements. Beef is a rich source of alpha-lipoic acid, as are broccoli and spinach. As a supplement, the usual dose is 100 to 200 mg daily.

Anti-aging secret:
undereating

We need food to live—all organisms do. But it doesn't follow that more food will make you live longer. In fact, it's quite the opposite. Research shows that undereating is an effective way to prolong life. The Chinese have always eaten moderately, and now a growing number of people worldwide are practicing calorie restriction, consuming approximately three-quarters of the typical calorie recommendation. Overeating stresses the body and increases its load of toxins. It's the fast track to the cemetery. Eating less keeps your metabolism in a more natural state, lowers LDL (bad) cholesterol and boosts HDL (good) cholesterol, keeps diabetes in check, regulates blood pressure, and optimizes cell division. When you restrict your food intake but pay attention to nutrition, your body becomes more efficient and effective, less burdened by the work of eliminating toxins. Eat small meals more frequently. Losing weight is the side effect in this case, not the main point. You are slowing down the aging process!

Chestnuts ward off winter flu

"Chestnuts roasting on an open fire . . ." evokes the European and U.S. tradition of enjoying this delicious nut in wintertime. Chestnuts have been popular in the Mediterranean region and Asia for centuries. Unlike other nuts, chestnuts are low in fat and high in fiber; they have a mild, sweet taste and a crumbly consistency. In China, the chestnut is known to be nourishing and tonic, an excellent aid during menopause, when your immune system weakens, leaving you more susceptible to disease. Chestnuts strengthen the kidney-adrenal system, bolster the immune system to ward off flu and fight infections, and offer plenty of protein to build you up. An excellent source of potassium, folate, and vitamins B6 and C, they are good roasted in the oven or cooked with chicken, lamb, beef, or pork as well as any dish with beans and legumes. Chestnut flour is also available for use in baking.

Eat food from your
own ecosystem

During your Second Spring, you want to eat organic, locally grown produce from farmers' markets and health food stores whenever possible. It's good for your health and good for the environment. Fresh, local fruits and vegetables contain more nutrients and are picked when naturally ripe. Commercial produce, on the other hand, is picked unripe, treated with ethylene gas to ripen artificially late, and shipped across the country on weeklong, sometimes monthlong, trips before it gets to your dinner table. (And think about the fuel used to transport it. What a waste!) Studies emerge regularly about the negative effects of pesticides and herbicides used on commercial crops: cancer risk, inflammation, and reproductive imbalance in humans and other animals. For health, vigor, and eco-kindness, choose food that grows close to home.

A healthy thymus = a vital you

The thymus is a fist-size gland located in the center of your chest, behind the sternum, that plays a crucial role in the functioning of the lymphatic and immune systems. It develops over time, peaking when you are around 30 or 35, then begins to physically diminish until, by age 70, it typically shrinks to the size of a pea. You experience the gland's waning as waning energy in your body. To help prevent this atrophying, the Chinese use astragalus root. Studies show it to be an *adaptogen*, meaning it corrects both high and low metabolic imbalances, acts on invaders wherever they attack the body, and promotes overall vitality. People can take 100 to 150 mg per day in capsules or drink astragalus tincture or tea. You can also use acupressure: With your index and middle finger, gently tap against the sternum (midway between the nipples) 50 times, morning and evening, to stimulate the thymus.

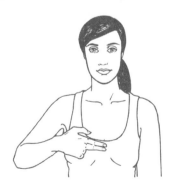

Up your immunity for an energy boost

You may not expect to have the same vim you had in your 20s, but do you find yourself looking at other energetic midlife women and wondering, "How can I be *this* tired?" In our practice, acupuncture has had good success in restoring the quality of life for many exhausted women. Acupuncture can modulate immune function, boosting it if low and calming it if overactive; we also use it to nourish the kidney-adrenal system to achieve healthy hormonal balance. You can build your immunity by eliminating foods that interfere with good health, such as dairy, alcohol, caffeine, sugar, and gluten-heavy foods like wheat and rye. At the same time, increase your intake of fresh fruits and vegetables, nuts and seeds, beans and legumes, and fish and poultry. Lastly, find a Chinese medicine doctor who can address energy problems with herbs and coach you on energy-enhancing exercises like tai chi and qi gong. Through these natural therapies, many women restore their former energy levels—and have a healthier lifestyle.

B tops A
in energy class

Fatigue can come from a deficiency of B vitamins. The B complex is important because it provides co-enzymes that aid in carbohydrate metabolism—and carbohydrates give your body energy. Many women don't get enough B vitamins, which are necessary to manufacture blood. It's possible to get all your Bs from eggs and fish (especially shellfish); sunflower, sesame, and other seeds; leafy green vegetables such as spinach and collard greens; and orange juice, among other dietary sources. Of particular importance are B6 and B12. Of course, you can also take B vitamins as a daily supplement; just be sure to take the whole B complex to avoid imbalance.

Walk away from
your energy slump

One simple way to improve your energy is to walk, but if you are not used to it or if you are ill, even walking can be an effort. If walking is difficult for you, I suggest you ease into a walking routine very gradually: Start small, and slowly increase the amount of time you walk. I usually begin by asking patients to walk 10 minutes a day for a week, and then increase it by five minutes every week. So on the second week you walk 15 minutes a day; the third week, 20, and so on, so that by the time you get to the fifth week, you are walking 30 minutes a day. You'll see an energy change around the end of the fourth week. The hardest part is getting started! If you are suffering from chronic illness and low energy, walking can build you up again, but you need to take that first step.

All that chive

A member of the garlic and onion family, Chinese chive (and all chives) has a very strong aroma. In America, it is usually used as flavoring, but it is more than just a seasoning. Throughout history, chives have been used for natural healing around the world because they contain a substantial amount of vitamin C, as well as essential minerals such as potassium, calcium, iron, and folic acid. In Chinese medicine, they are used to clear stuffy noses, prevent bad breath, ease stomachaches, and strengthen the kidney-adrenal system. Additionally, chives strengthen the lower back and improve poor circulation that gives you cold hands and feet. I recommend eating chives as a vegetable, chopped and stir-fried, or mixing chopped chives with ground chicken or turkey to stuff ravioli or dumplings. You'll find large bunches at Asian markets and health food stores.

Spice up your
mental vitality

Hazardous condition: brain fog! Most of us experience it intermittently, but it tends to become more frequent around midlife. To stay alert, you'll be tempted to reach for that cup of coffee—but wait a minute. Coffee will give you a jolt, all right, but it will also produce a letdown when it wears off, deplete the calcium in your system, and over-stimulate the kidneys, all of which ultimately robs your body of vital energy. Next time you need a boost, go to your spice cabinet instead. Many natural herbs and spices offer gentler, healthier alternatives. Make a tea from mint, lemon balm, cinnamon, oregano, dill, cilantro, rosemary, bay leaves, sage, coriander, fennel, anise, basil, or garlic. All contain vital chemicals that stimulate alertness, in the volatile oils that give them their fragrance and delicious taste. Let them spice up your energy and keep your brain humming.

Life's a marathon— keep score with the glycemic index

What, another statistic to learn about your health? Don't worry. This one is simple, and very important. The *glycemic index* is a measurement of how quickly the food you eat converts to glucose, the substance your body needs for energy. Foods with a high glycemic index (HGI) give you a quick rush, but fatigue soon follows when your blood sugar drops. The secret to steady, robust energy lies in low glycemic index (LGI) foods. Bread, pasta, baked potatoes, and carrots are all HGI, as are most refined grains. An athlete competing in a 100-yard sprint would eat a high-glycemic meal for quick energy before the race—but most of us are not running a 100-yard dash. Our lives are more like marathons; we need to pace ourselves. LGI foods include grains such as barley, bulgur, quinoa, and amaranth, as well as peanuts, most nuts and seeds, beans and legumes, and of course chicken, fish, and meat. For smooth and steady energy keep an eye on your food's glycemic index.

Metabolic mover:
chromium

What happens when your body digests food? Metabolic processes break it down into glucose and other nutrients. Insulin is produced in your body, which then signals the cells to open their doors. But things don't stop there. You need chromium to move the sugar molecule through the door. Without chromium, people develop either too much blood sugar, resulting in diabetes, or too little, which causes low blood sugar. The average American diet provides only 15 mcg of chromium, although the recommended daily intake is 120 mcg. To bridge the gap, sprinkle brewer's yeast, the natural substance used to ferment beer, into your power shakes, or add it to your baked goods. Black pepper is another good source, ground onto compatible foods. Cinnamon, clove, and ginger all contain good amounts of chromium, as does broccoli. In supplement form, the suggested dose is up to 200 mcg a day.

Protein for lunch
wards off energy slump

If you have a hard time staying awake in the afternoon, you're not alone. Many people feel suddenly drowsy a few hours after lunch, usually because lunch consists largely of carbohydrates, which burn very quickly, leaving you without enough energy to last until dinner. Make sure you eat a light lunch that has about 4 ounces of protein—about the size of a pack of cards. Proteins have a low glycemic index, so they burn slowly and provide steady fuel lasting two to four hours. This gives you a steady supply of the glucose you need throughout the workday. A piece of chicken, turkey, or fish with a salad is an excellent lunch. Skip the bread, pasta, rice, potato—and don't eat sweets at lunchtime. If your energy wanes in the afternoon, eat a piece of fruit, some hummus, or even a cup of instant soup for a snack to feed your metabolism without overloading yourself with calories.

Ginseng, the herbal superhero

In capsules or as tea, ginseng root can pick you up when you're tired without inducing that hyper, frazzled energy you get from stimulants like caffeine. In China, people are willing to pay thousands of dollars for 10-year-old ginseng, which is even more potent. Traditionally, ginseng is used to stimulate the libido, but the herb contains phytoestrogens useful in supporting hormonal balance and has been classified as an adaptogen, meaning that it helps the immune system to withstand stress from the environment. It also possesses antioxidant and anticancer properties. Ginseng is an indispensable herb for women at any age, and in particular for women in menopause and afterward. Traditionally, ginseng is used to stimulate the libido. A daily dose of 300 mg can help keep hormones in balance and can subtly improve sex drive. It is widely available in health food stores, at naturopaths' offices, and online, as a single product or as part of a revitalizing formula with other Chinese herbs.

Yellow boosts your energy wattage

In our culture we say we're feeling "blue" if we're down in the dumps, "in the pink" if we are happy—and these aren't just figures of speech. Colors matter! Studies show that color waves send impulses to the pituitary and pineal glands in the brain, which control energy and mood. Different colors affect us emotionally and physically. According to research, the color yellow and its various shades—from lemon to mustard to saffron to amber—are the most energizing of all the colors. Does that give you a few ideas? Paint your room yellow, put on a bright yellow outfit, brighten up your kitchen with a yellow lampshade, switch to a yellow screen saver. Power your own energy with the color of the sun.

Inulin for your
inner ecosystem

As you age, you probably notice that food does not move through your system the way it used to and you have more frequent bloating, irregularity, or gas. This is usually because the microflora, or helpful bacteria that line your digestive tract, have become scant or out of balance. A certain kind of dietary fiber can help. The natural substance inulin (not to be confused with insulin) serves as a *prebiotic*, an agent that is not digested but energizes beneficial bacteria in the system and inhibits detrimental ones. Like other prebiotic fibers, inulin eases constipation. But while most stimulate growth and activity of good bacteria in the stomach and upper intestines and then run out of steam, inulin continues to be active all the way to the colon, which tends to have the worst imbalances. Good sources of inulin include chicory root, dandelion root, Jerusalem artichoke, apples, and bananas. In supplement form, the typical dose is 2 grams with meals.

The midlife woman's great date

The jujube date has been used since ancient times as a tonifying nutrient, a blood cleanser, and an important herbal adjunct to other tonics, especially in combination with ginseng and dong quai, or Chinese angelica. It comes in two varieties differentiated by their color: Black jujube is considered an energy tonic; red jujube is used as a blood tonic. In China, jujube dates are eaten as a tasty dried fruit. Cooked in chicken soup or brewed as tea, the date is a medicinal aid to people suffering from fatigue or chronic illness and to mothers after giving birth. For women over 40, it will rebuild blood by stimulating kidney and bone marrow functions and will increase energy, soothe the mind, and balance the hormones. Jujube dates can be found in Asian markets, select health food stores, and online.

Is anemia
dragging you down?

As a woman, you are prone to anemia in your prime, when you need to make menstrual blood, but also later, when stress and sometimes medications take their toll. Low iron also leads to anemia, which is characterized by fatigue and lack of energy. The cure, of course, is to get iron in your diet. Iron-rich foods include dried plums and all the leafy green vegetables: collard greens, Swiss chard, kale, mustard greens, parsley, beet greens. Vitamin C helps the absorption of iron, so squeeze lemon juice on your salad. Other nutrients critical for blood production are folic acid, found in many leafy greens as well as papaya, mung beans, and adzuki beans; and of course B12, available only from animal products like eggs, chicken, and red meat. Keep in mind that tannin—found in coffee or tea—interferes with iron absorption, so make sure you don't drink coffee or tea with your iron-rich foods. Unless you have a confirmed case of iron deficiency, I don't suggest taking iron supplements, which are constipating. Try to get your iron from your food. Overcome your anemia, and your energy will rebound!

Plums juice up your energy and health

One of the most popular health foods in China and Japan is the plum, fresh or in its dried form, also called prunes. Plums are consumed as snacks and breakfast foods, added to sauces, and even used as medicine. Most often eaten dried, they are sometimes pickled with salt and vinegar. Used therapeutically, dried plum is prized for its energy-boosting properties. This may be due to its abundance of antioxidant phytonutrients called *phenols* and its ability to increase iron absorption into the body. Iron raises the level of hemoglobin in the blood, which in turn helps to oxygenate cells. For athletes and other active people, there is no better energizing food than dried plums, which provide glucose to muscle cells at an even, steady pace and are packed with essential minerals like potassium and magnesium. They are an excellent snack for weight management. The dried sour plum is used in Chinese medicine to treat digestion problems, allergies, and parasites. There are three main producers of plums worldwide: China, Russia, and the United States, where 99 percent of domestic dried plums come from a single state, California. Next time you want to juice up your energy, pack some prunes to go.

A whiff of jasmine jazzes you up

Just as exercise, diet, and supplements improve health and vitality, certain smells can energize you. Aromas can alter your mood, even your actions. Studies show that different smells affect brain waves, which of course help determine your energy patterns. Perfumers and smart marketers have been using odors to change consumer behavior for years. Different smells bring about different results. Jasmine, for instance, stimulates the beta waves in the frontal lobe of your brain, which are associated with alertness. Next time you need a little energy, take a whiff of jasmine: Put a dab of its essential oil on your temples, or inhale deeply the steam from that cup of jasmine tea. A natural energy boost from a flower!

Chinese herbs for heart health: the big 5

Many midlife women develop plaque buildup in their arteries, especially the coronary arteries, due to loss of elasticity in the blood vessels and a natural increase in cholesterol. Follow your cardiologist's recommended protocols—and discuss using nature's help, too, with the herbs in this traditional Chinese formula:

1) **Ginseng** reduces cholesterol and has shown positive effects on blood vessel elasticity.

2) **Dong quai,** or Chinese angelica root, is traditionally used to treat blockages and help increase blood flow.

3) **Sacred pine** contains a potent antioxidant called *picnogenol* in its bark, needles, and nut that helps reduce inflammation in the blood vessels, lowering the risk of plaque buildup.

4) **Ginkgo** also increases microcapillary circulation and expands blood vessels.

5) **Hawthorn berries** reduce fat and mucus accumulation, purify the blood, and improve blood flow.

These herbs are available separately or as a combined supplement from Chinese pharmacies and in some health food stores. Some of the herbs, like ginkgo, possess mild blood-thinning properties and may interact with blood-thinning drugs. You must talk to your medical doctor and cardiologist before you take these herbs if you are already taking prescription medications.

The healthy
Rise-and-shine ritual

Busy as you are all week, you may feel you've earned the right to sleep late on weekends. But are you really doing yourself a favor? Your body functions best with routine and rhythm—sleeping in actually throws off your body clock and ends up making you tired. There is an art to waking up and it's not hard to learn how to program your brain to activate your body's energy in the morning. I call my three-step wake-up routine for high energy "The Three S's": Stretch, Strengthen, and Step. When you wake up, before you do anything else, stretch in bed: Pull your knees up to your chest and perform other simple stretches, whatever feels good. Then strengthen your muscles by doing some abdominal crunches, raising your legs. Finally, step out of bed and keep on stepping—take a walk first thing, before your shower, breakfast, or any other morning activity. Try it and you will wake up refreshed and have consistent energy throughout the day.

CHAPTER 4

Enhance Brain Power,
Hearing, and Eyesight

YOUR BRAIN CAN TAKE YOU on an emotional roller-coaster ride. You
may have felt blue just before your period, or experienced the forget-
fulness of pregnancy brain, perhaps followed by postpartum depression
and related cognitive changes. At age forty and afterward, women
often complain of a sort of fogginess, which is especially worrisome
to those with family histories of senility or Alzheimer's. Common reports
among our female patients at Tao of Wellness include things like
being unable to remember the name of the person they met the night
before or what they went to get in the grocery store aisle, or difficulty
concentrating on tasks like balancing a checkbook. These symptoms
can occur at any age, but often occur at midlife, along with vision and
hearing decline, but when you understand the underlying reasons and
use appropriate natural remedies, you can prevent or reverse brain
aging and sensory deterioration.

A change in mental acuity doesn't have to signal the beginning
of declining brain function. Often it reflects physiological swings in
the brain associated with hormonal changes, the effects of emotional
stress, or reactions to environmental toxins like pesticides or heavy
metals. A mild slowing of memory and thought typically occurs
because aging lowers levels of chemical neurotransmitters, the mes-
sengers that relay information from one neuron to the next. Emotional
trauma and stress reduce blood flow to the brain and stimulate
production of the hormone cortisol, which in large amounts is toxic
to nerve cells. Circulation also comes into play, as plaque narrows
blood vessels, reducing blood flow to the brain, eyes, and ears. In this
chapter, I provide suggestions that can increase your brain function,

reduce stress naturally, and boost your body's hormone-production capabilities with nutrients, herbal supplements, acupressure, and meditation and other mind-body practices.

Your Brain's Relation to Hormones, Stress, and Toxins

Hormones have intimate connections to proper brain function. Starting in the early 40s, the female brain becomes less sensitive to the monthly surges of estrogen and progesterone caused by the menstrual cycle. As you approach menopause, your ovaries' production of estrogen decreases and the output of the adrenal glands, which produce most of your androgen and testosterone, also drops precipitously. Estrogen affects many aspects of a woman's cognitive health, including maintaining blood flow to the brain, balancing neurotransmitters, and protecting the brain from shrinking with age. Testosterone, on the other hand, is involved in mental acuity, sexual arousal, and muscle strength. The areas of brain shrinkage most noticeable with aging include regions for concentration, memory, judgment, decision-making, and emotional processing. Changing levels and sensitivity to estrogen around menopause can cause fluctuations in dopamine, serotonin, and acetylcholine, which can bring about memory and mood disorders. Natural ways to boost your own hormone production are found throughout the book.

Prolonged stress can damage the hippocampus, an area of the brain that is important for memory. Studies show that continued stress diminishes replacement of brain cells and causes dendrites to wither in the hippocampus; the stress hormone cortisol, when released in excess, actually causes shrinkage of the hippocampus. Insufficient levels of the neurotransmitter serotonin may also aggravate brain aging—when serotonin levels are increased, cells in the hippocampus regenerate. The good news is that stress response can be counteracted through stress-reduction techniques like meditation, tai chi, and biofeedback. More and more studies are refining our comprehension of neuroplasticity—the capacity of certain brain areas to regenerate or compensate for other damaged areas by taking over their functions. Mind-body training techniques can help heal the brain and keep it strong. You will find some of them throughout this chapter.

As modern standards of living have improved, our species has also generated toxins that now overrun our environment and threaten our own existence. These range from pesticides in food to everyday plastics that contaminate everything they come in contact with, to heavy metals in water and soil, to drugs we take for our ailments. Even though our bodies possess a blood-brain barrier designed to protect our cognitive command center from toxic assaults, the negative effects of environmental poisons on brain function have been well documented. High levels of lead and mercury cause brain damage; less well known is that monosodium glutamate (MSG), artificial colors, and preservatives can disrupt proper brain function, affecting focus and concentration. Besides trying to avoid these substances in your everyday life, periodic cleansing is useful to aid your body's natural detoxification processes.

Chinese Medicine's View of Healthy Cognitive, Visual, and Auditory Performance

The health of your kidneys and heart is key to a healthy brain. According to Chinese medicine, the kidney network performs multiple jobs, regulating aspects of brain function such as memory as well as the hormonal system, reproductive system, hearing, head hair, and health of the bones and marrow. The heart network is responsible for the delivery of nutrients to the brain and elimination of waste products. The heart network is also the house of the spirit or consciousness that directs the brain in its various cognitive activities. When both organ networks are functioning optimally and in harmony, you experience clarity of mind, sharpness of recall, and peaceful contentment. Acupuncture and Chinese herbal therapy target the kidneys and heart and often yield improved brain performance. In addition, vitality-boosting mind-body exercises like tai chi and qi gong have been found to enhance cognitive functions.

Due to wear and tear, vision and hearing often decline with time. To a certain degree this is normal, but much of the quality of our lives is determined by these two crucial senses, through which we receive input from the world around us. Age-related degeneration of the eyes, including cataracts, glaucoma, and macular degeneration, should be taken very seriously. Likewise, loss of hearing is a grave handicap and should be addressed immediately. The various causes of declining vision and hearing range from diminished circulation to the eyes and ears, a buildup of toxins in the body, and environmental damage from things like UV radiation and noise pollution. Chinese medicine recognizes all these factors and additionally correlates vision and hearing loss with weakness in the liver and kidney networks.

Act now to prevent eye and ear problems by drinking parsley juice, taking ginkgo supplements, and using acupressure that targets your eyes and ears. But if you're having trouble seeing or hearing, Chinese medicine can help with remedies, including herbal and acupuncture therapies, that fortify and support the liver and kidneys. In this chapter, you'll find natural ways to stimulate your brain's regenerative powers and bring your life to a higher level of performance and fulfillment.

Green tea helps fend off Alzheimer's

In China and Japan, aging doesn't seem to mean inevitable cognitive decline, and when it does occur it is often less severe than the syndrome seen in the West. The explanation for this disparity isn't geography. There is evidence that green tea may actually ward off Alzheimer's disease and other forms of mental degeneration. Green tea is filled with antioxidants called *polyphenols*, which have been shown to increase cognitive acuity and learning ability. The effects are attributed to one polyphenol in particular, catechin. Green tea contains over four times the concentration of catechins found in black tea. Why? Researchers aren't sure, but the minimal processing associated with green tea may help to preserve a higher concentration of the antioxidants. If you replace that morning cup of coffee with green tea, you get more than a momentary pickup—you'll reap long-term benefits for your brain.

Memory snack:
a nibble for your noodle

Nature is full of wonderful foods that nourish your brain, but in your busy life, have you taken the time to find out what they are? And if you do know, do you find it hard to fit them into your diet? I decided to make it easy for my patients—and you—by listing the following wonder foods as snacks to nibble on throughout the day. You can also put together a batch of **Dr. Mao's Anti-aging Brain Mix** using all these ingredients:

- 1 cup walnut
- $1/2$ cup pine nuts
- $1/4$ cup sesame seeds
- $1/2$ cup pumpkin seeds
- $1/3$ cup of dried goji berries (found in health food stores)
- $1/2$ cup dried apricots
- $1/2$ cup of dried blueberries

Mix the ingredients evenly and pack in a sealed container or zipper bag to preserve freshness. Eat a small handful between meals every day as a snack. This mix of nuts and fruits supplies essential fatty acids, carotenoids, and antioxidants that will maintain a steady supply of fuel and energy for your brain.

Big brain help
from little fish

Don't be one of those people who turns up her nose at anchovies and sardines—you'd be missing out on the brain benefits that these little fish offer! *Dimethyl-amino-ethanol* (DMAE), a nutrient found in anchovies and sardines, is a precursor to the amino acid choline and neurotransmitter acetylcholine. Unlike choline itself, DMAE can pass through the blood/brain barrier to fire up the cholinergic nervous system. For people with declining levels of acetylcholine in the brain, this proccess is believed to improve concentration and mood. Studies have shown that DMAE promotes increased daytime energy, focus, and concentration as well as deeper sleep at night among healthy individuals. Athletes use it to bolster strength and speed. And if that weren't enough, DMAE has been found to be a powerful membrane stabilizer that reverses age spots on the skin. So don't snub these little swimmers— they're good for your brain and keep those age spots away.

Nutritional "cocktail"
that goes to your head

Certain nutrients like vitamin C, carotenoids, trace minerals, amino acids, and lecithin have all been shown to be essential nutrients for healthy brain function. For those of you who'd enjoy getting all this in one beverage you can drink every day, here's the recipe for **Dr. Mao's Brain Tonic**:

- $1/2$ cup of fresh or dried apricot
- 1 teaspoon of fresh lemon juice
- $1/2$ teaspoon of kelp powder
- 1 organic egg yolk

Blend these ingredients into one cup of soy milk or goat milk. If you're using dried apricots, soak them in water first to reconstitute. Drink the blended mixture cold, one glass every day. You'll see the difference when you give your brain the nutrition it needs.

Healthy fats make you
one smart cookie

Low-fat diets keep you slim, but take a toll on hormonal health. Fats are an important part of your body's makeup; essential fatty acids (the good fats) are responsible for optimum health of skin, joints, the immune and hormonal systems, and especially the brain. Women who have low reserves of fat often have scant menstrual periods or none at all, a sign of low estrogen and progesterone. This may lead to bone loss and a host of other premature aging conditions, including cognitive decline. Ideally, your body fat should amount to 21 to 35 percent of total body weight. Get healthy fats from oils derived from vegetables, nuts, and seeds. My favorites include flaxseed, almond, walnut, sesame, and olive oils. Use generous amounts with your vegetables, salads, beans, and whole grain dishes. Eat foods filled with healthy fats, such as cold-water fish, nuts and seeds, avocados, and olives.

A diet to remember, in more ways than one!

If your parents insisted that you eat your broccoli, they were looking out for your intelligence. It's one of the foods high in *choline*, an essential nutrient for memory and brain health. Choline is a precursor to the neurotransmitter acetylcholine, which contributes to the efficiency of brain processes. Our bodies produce choline in the liver for use by the brain, but as we age, natural choline output declines, and its neurochemical action becomes weaker and less efficient. Research has shown that taking choline supplements of up to 1,200 mg per day can improve the production of acetylcholine, enhancing cognitive ability and boosting memory power. I always recommend starting with good dietary sources, in this case eggs, soybeans, black beans, kidney beans, peanuts, cabbage, and cruciferous vegetables like cauliflower, Brussels sprouts, and, of course, that broccoli you didn't want to eat when you were a kid. Maybe now you'll change your mind—and your memory.

Chinese moss fights memory loss

In recent years, Western medicine has become aware of a nutrient extracted from Chinese club moss that helps to improve learning, memory retrieval, and memory retention. The moss, *Huperzia serrata*, yields a substance called Huperzine A that is similar to drugs used to control Alzheimer's disease. Research has revealed that this natural alkaloid inhibits the breakdown of *acetylcholine*, a neurochemical directly involved in memory and awareness—exactly what the pharmaceuticals do. The Chinese have used it to boost memory and treat inflammation, fever, and even schizophrenia. It is usually brewed as tea and administered at a dose of one or two cups per day. If your health food store or Asian grocery does not stock the moss itself—which you can steep in hot water, one teaspoon per cup, and drink as tea twice a day—it is also available in capsule form; the recommended dose is 50 mcg twice a day. Because of its potent actions, you should only take Huperzine A under the supervision of your doctor.

This is your brain
on herbs

For thousands of years, Chinese traditional medicine has used three particular herbs as brain tonics and to help prevent loss of mental function with age. Sage has been shown to increase oxygen to the brain cortex and to help improve concentration. Mugwort, long known in Asian culture as a warming herb that opens the channels and increases blood and energy flow, dilates capillaries, boosts circulation, and improves delivery of nutrients. Rosemary contains volatile oils that help stimulate brain activities and increase brain alertness. You can easily incorporate all three herbs into your diet: Sage and rosemary are excellent flavorings for poultry dishes and soups; mugwort, available in health food stores, can be added to your salad. You can combine all three herbs to make tea—one heaping teaspoon of each in a cup of hot water, steeped for five minutes. Drink three cups a day to keep your brain humming.

B12 for a
brain boost

If perimenopause or menopause gives you brain fog, you
may be deficient in B12. The vitamin plays many important
roles in the body, from maintaining red blood cell production and normal nervous system function to metabolizing
protein and fats. Studies have also shown that people
with higher B12 levels in their blood performed better on
mental tests than those with less. An estimated 10 percent
or more of people over 60 are deficient in this particular
vitamin. B12 deficiency often leads to anemia and various
nervous system dysfunctions. You can get plenty of B12
in your diet from eggs, fish, and meat, preferably organic.
Vegans can take a daily supplement of 500 mcg in capsule
form or, even better, a sublingual preparation that dissolves
under the tongue. If you're perimenopausal or menopausal,
the typical dosage is up to 1,000 mg every day.

Remember this today, and you won't forget tomorrow

We often take our memory for granted until it starts acting up. Then we panic: Where are those car keys? What if this keeps happening? For those with a family history of Alzheimer's disease, these incidents are of particular concern. A simple amino acid can help. Daily supplements of 2 grams a day of the amino acid L-carnitine can slow the onset of mental deterioration, according to research. L-carnitine is found chiefly in the heart and skeletal muscles. Its main job is to carry fatty acids through cell membranes to the mitochondrion—the cell's engine—which uses them as cellular energy. Brain tissue also holds a rich supply of L-carnitine. Even when you have plenty of those wonderful omega fatty acids, if your L-carnitine level is low, your brain and muscles can't use them. The sole dietary source of this amino acid is meat, but vegetarians may find it worthwhile to take supplements to help fight the onset of age-related memory loss.

A little help "upstairs"

Popular in Asia for its many anti-aging properties, *shou wu* (also called *fo-ti* or *polygonum root*) has two beneficial effects "upstairs"—on your head and your hair. Studies show that the herb helps you maintain a healthy memory thanks to its antioxidant and anti-inflammatory properties. Shou wu is also known to restore hair growth and reverse graying. Rich in vitamin E and the B-complex vitamins, shou wu normalizes estrogen profiles in women, raises blood production, boosts immune function, maintains healthy cholesterol levels, and promotes intestinal regularity. It is a common ingredient in herbal anti-aging formulas found in health food stores, online, or at the offices of acupuncturists and herbalists.

Brain fuel from under the sea

Throughout the ages people have sought magic substances that will keep mental faculties intact throughout a long life. Leaves like ginkgo biloba and roots like ginseng have proven to have some real effects, but it turns out that the powerhouse brain aid comes from the sea. Microalgae from the ocean and uncontaminated lakes, such as chorella, blue green algae, spirulina, seaweed, and kelp, are high-protein, high-energy, easy-to-digest supplements that support healthy brain function and contain more than a hundred trace minerals, a bounty unmatched by anything that grows on land. Microalgae are usually available in your health food store in several forms that are simple to incorporate into your diet—powders you dissolve in juice or flakes you can sprinkle on salads, for example—to help you sail through menopause with the brain power you need.

Good for the muscles, good for the brain

Even if you are not an athlete, chances are you'll benefit from buffing up on one of bodybuilders' favorite amino acids. *L-glutamine*, popular among nutritionists and athletes, helps to minimize breakdown of muscle tissue after physical exertion, meaning anything from bench-pressing 250 pounds to going to your aerobics class. But that's not all—it crosses the blood/brain barrier and becomes *glutamic acid*, a potent brain fuel. We can all use that! L-glutamine also helps maintain normal levels of growth hormone and regulates blood sugar. Dietary sources of L-glutamine include animal proteins such as beef, pork, poultry, and yogurt and vegetables such as raw spinach, raw parsley, and cabbage. As a supplement it may be swallowed in capsule form or taken in a sublingual (under-the-tongue) preparation. The typical recommended dose is 2 to 3 grams a day, although serious bodybuilders use up to 30 grams. Eat glutamine-rich foods listed above or take L-glutamine and other supplements along with your meals.

L-theanine leaves you **calm, not drowsy**

When you feel wired or overstimulated, you may pour a drink or pop a tranquilizer to chill out—only to find that you've slowed your mental functioning as well. You may become drowsy at work, or start to make bad decisions. There's a better way. A natural amino acid, *L-theanine*, promotes relaxation with none of these negative side effects. L-theanine can stimulate the production of alpha waves in the brain, producing feelings of calmness and well-being without reducing focus. Because it crosses the blood/brain barrier, it can increase levels of the neurotransmitter dopamine, which benefits mood while actually improving learning and concentration. The amino acid also has antioxidant properties that support healthy cardiovascular function and immune reactions; a blood pressure regulator, it can ease the stress and tension associated with PMS. How do you get this little mood miracle? It is found almost exclusively in green tea. If supplements work better for you, the usual suggested dose is 100 mg daily.

Brain fade—is it midlife or your meds?

In the West, we come to assume that certain changes we experience in our 40s—brain fade, for example—are symptoms of the midlife transition. But common medications can cause memory loss and temporary confusion. Painkillers and cold medications that contain diphenhydramine, such as Benadryl and Tylenol PM, may create these temporary brain lapses. If you have high blood pressure, you may be taking methyldopa (Aldomet, by its commercial name) or propranolol (commercial name Inderal), which can adversely affect memory. Brain fog can occur with tricyclic antidepressants such as amitriptyline (commercial name Elavil). Make a list of the medications you are taking, and consult your doctor if you are experiencing sudden memory loss, or concentration problems, or mental confusion. If these pharmaceuticals are implicated, you can also see a naturopath or acupuncturist to explore natural alternatives and discuss them with your physician.

Three ways to keep
brain decline at bay

You can take action now to prevent decline in brain function. Most of the time, loss of memory and cognitive function is due to plaque buildup and diminished blood supply to the brain, which compromise the delivery of nutrients and oxygen. To help prevent this, engage in cardiovascular exercise on a regular basis starting now, to a heart rate of 120 beats per minute for half an hour, at least five times a week. The Chinese herb ginkgo biloba, traditionally used to increase focus and concentration, also increases blood flow to the microcapillaries in your brain and other organs, and fights free radicals that damage your cells. You can brew ginkgo tea or take in supplement form. A typical dosage is 120 mg daily. (If you are taking medications, consult your doctor before taking ginkgo.) And don't forget to give your brain a workout by trying new things. Learn a new language, dance step, or musical instrument—being an amateur keeps you young!

Lefty or righty, try the other side

Some people seem to maintain perfect mental function throughout their lives. No single explanation fits every case, but challenging the brain with brand-new tasks improves capacity in younger people, and it also has a restorative effect for mental faculties that are declining. To start buffing up your brain power right now, practice performing everyday activities with your nondominant hand. If you're right-handed, use your left hand to eat, comb your hair, brush your teeth. Use a pen to write your name, then practice writing more and pick up speed. Put your mouse pad on the other side of the keyboard. All these changes stimulate communication between the two hemispheres of the brain and improve mental capacity as well as physical balance. Tai chi also coaches people to use the right and left side of the body equally. Try it in sports: If you play tennis, switch the racquet to your other hand and play with the nondominant side.

Use it
or lose it

Think of your brain as a muscle: It gets stronger with exercise. Your everyday mental tasks are like walking, but now it's time for a real workout. Mental exercise can include games like crossword puzzles and chess or memorizing names, shopping lists, phone numbers—as long as it's something new to you. The key to success is to do it on a regular basis. For example, when I was young, my father had us memorize Tang dynasty poetry. Each day we had to memorize a new poem and recite it back. You could learn the words to a new song. Be sure you practice every day at the same time; you are developing and activating new neural pathways, and consistent cycles will keep the brain on track. Keep challenging yourself with new tasks. How about setting aside the calculator and adding manually instead? Try it!

Finger exercise for brain agility

Many people marvel that Asian children seem so smart. It may be because they use their fingers more often. They eat with chopsticks at home and they used to compute with an abacus in school; in fact, some studies have been done with children who use the abacus daily and findings show that engaging the fingers stimulates nerve endings that go directly to the brain, increasing circulation. You can take advantage of this to keep your brain in tune. Your Second Spring is a great time to practice motor activities that use your fingertips, like crocheting, knitting, and other arts and crafts; manipulating small puzzles; and playing the piano or a stringed instrument. For an exercise you can do anywhere, at any time, put one finger on top of the one next to it, then try to stack the next finger on top of that. Or hold a pencil or pen between your index and middle fingers, roll it over until it's held between the middle and ring fingers, then again to between the ring finger and pinky.

Good point!
Acupressure for the brain

According to traditional Chinese medicine, the kidney-adrenal system provides the energy necessary for healthy brain functions, so it's no surprise that the acupoint used to stimulate memory and concentration is located on the kidney meridian. You can perform acupressure on yourself by stimulating the kidney meridian point, called Kidney-3, located between the Achilles tendon and the ankle bone on the inside of your foot. Chinese practitioners of acupuncture and acupressure utilize this point to strengthen kidney function, increase mental clarity, improve memory, help the lower back, and restore vitality and libido. To activate the energy channel to your brain, pinch the point with your thumb and index finger for one minute, then release. Pinch again for one minute. Do this for three to five minutes as needed. You'll notice results almost immediately and receive better results cumulatively after doing it daily for two weeks.

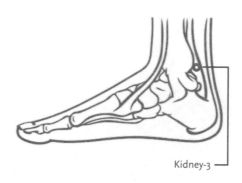

Kidney-3

To solve problems, color them gone

In Chinese medicine, all animate and inanimate things are categorized according to their energy type, or elemental type. Each element is associated with a particular color. For someone engaged in the mental task of problem-solving, each color has different attributes: White is all about fact finding, gathering information; red concerns how you feel about the facts; yellow is for finding the opportunity or upside to them; green brainstorms the most creative solution to the problem; and finally blue/black gives insight on the downside or worst-case scenario. Take pens of different colors and write out these five attributes on paper. Visually absorb the color vibration of each. When you are in one of these stages of problem-solving, consider surrounding yourself with the appropriate color, or wearing it. Sit in a room with walls painted yellow to see the bright side, or a green room to generate answers. Let the Chinese elemental colors help you think.

Dietary tips to
perk up your ears

As you hit middle age, reduced blood flow to the ears, hardening of the tiny bone that vibrates to transmit sound waves (*otosclerosis*), degeneration of the seashell-like structure in the inner ear (the *cochlea*), blood pressure medication, and damage from infections can impair your hearing. Luckily, there are natural ways to improve your hearing function. First and foremost, be sure you eat a diet rich in vitamin A and C as well as the B complex, especially niacin and folic acid. That means fish, carrots, citrus, asparagus, parsley, and other leafy green vegetables. If this is impossible for you, take daily supplements. A traditional remedy for improving hearing is to prepare a drink using raw garlic and onions. Put the garlic and onions in a blender with a little warm water and buzz. Strain out the pulp and keep the juice. Drink about two ounces a day for a month.

Herbal
hearing aid

Chinese tradition holds that the body is animated by a vital essence that keeps us vigorous and healthy. When it is depleted by overwork, stress, or trauma—and who hasn't experienced one or more of these by midlife?—the result is a deficiency that can lead to premature decline in your sensory faculties, including hearing. Factors that can diminish acuity in our hearing over the years include excess anger, frustration, and bouts of flu and other viruses. The traditional Chinese remedy is a tea made from herbs that gently restore the ear.

My recipe:

• 1 heaping tablespoon each of cilantro, oregano, rosemary, sage, and cinnamon
• 3 slices fresh ginger
• 4 cups water

Boil for 15 minutes, then strain. Fresh herbs are always preferred, but dried will work, too. Make sure to cover the pan during boiling to prevent the volatile oils from escaping. Drink three cups a day for at least three weeks to see results.

The buzz on hearing loss: what not to do

As you age, you'll want to keep your ears covered—healthwise, that is! To guard against hearing loss, take a look at your daily habits. Did you know that drinking a lot of coffee increases your chance of hearing loss? Caffeine reduces the blood flow to the ears, so make sure you limit yourself to one 8-ounce cup of coffee a day. Better yet, drink decaf. Be sure it has been decaffeinated using a water process rather than harsh chemicals. You can decaffeinate tea by steeping it for 45 seconds, pouring off the water, then adding fresh water to the teabag. The fresh cup will have only 25 percent of the caffeine. A high-cholesterol diet is also bad for your hearing, because plaque buildup affects the arteries that serve the auditory nerves. Reduce your intake of saturated fat. Nicotine too diminishes blood flow to the nerves, and also interferes with the healing of small capillaries injured by loud noise. In fact, studies show that smokers have more hearing loss when exposed to noise than their nonsmoking co-workers.

Eardrops, not Q-tips

People commonly think they should clean their ears with a Q-tip—wrong! This is one of the worst things you can do because it introduces bacteria into the ear canal and pushes earwax deeper. Fingers are just as bad. Earwax is normal and healthy, serving to protect your eardrum from bacteria, dust, and water. Unless the wax is obstructing your ear canal, leave it alone. If it does form a blockage, use an over-the-counter earwax removal kit containing drops to soften the wax so it dissolves naturally. Alternatively, an ear specialist can wash the ear canal for you. Chinese herbalists make eardrops out of mullein flower, which is available in American health food stores. To make your own, soak 2 ounces of the crushed dried flower in 4 ounces of olive oil for two weeks, and then strain through a cheesecloth. I recommend to my patients that they put one drop of the oil in each ear daily for one week. After using the oil, massage the ear front and back by placing your middle finger in front of the ear and your index finger behind it, and stroking it up and down vigorously.

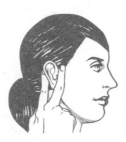

Massage away deafness

During menopause, as endocrine function declines, the microcapillaries feeding your auditory nerves harden and lose their elasticity, decreasing blood circulation to the inner ear. Calcium deposits may also accumulate, affecting the way the vibrating bone in your ear transmits sound. Many women complain that they are gradually losing their hearing or developing a ringing in their ears. But you can be proactive to prevent or reverse these changes. The traditional Chinese technique is to use cupping massage. Place your palms over your ears, closing them completely, with your fingers pointing toward the back of your head. While they are cupped, drum the back of your skull with your fingers 50 times. Then, with your hands cupping your ears, suddenly release them to pop the pressure in your ears. The pressure is low enough to do no damage to your ear, but high enough to open up the ear canal and Eustachian tube. Do this about 10 times. Now place your index fingers in the crevice right behind your earlobes and massage the area in a small circular motion 50 times. Repeat this traditional practice twice a day, morning and evening.

Decibel attack!
Protect your ears

Just as you'd protect any other part of your body from the danger of injury with padding or a helmet, you need to protect your ears from excessive noise. Exposure to loud noise is the second-biggest contributing factor to hearing loss—aging is the first. So take precautions. To protect your hearing from being damaged by loud movies or concerts, buy earplugs. You can carry them with you and use them anywhere. Make sure the earplugs have a rating of 15, which means that they reduce noise by 15 decibels. If you want superprotection, you can go to your ear specialist or audiologist and get custom-made earplugs that can reduce noise levels by about 35 decibels. Then go out dancing! Even if you end up right next to a speaker, you're prepared.

Look alive!
Eye care for midlife

More older people wear glasses than young ones, but diminished eyesight is not an inevitable part of living long. Take these steps to promote and preserve the health of your eyes.

1) The UV rays that harm the skin can also damage your eyes, so be sure to wear sunglasses on bright sunny days.

2) Eat like a visionary! Your diet should include at least three servings of antioxidant-rich foods such as spinach, carrots, and squash every day. Between meals, snack on goji berries.

3) Add to your daily vitamins a supplement called *lutein*, a plant carotenoid that aids eye health. Ginkgo biloba, best known for promoting brain function, also improves vision. You'll find both of these in health food stores.

4) When your eyes feel tired, lie down and place slices of cucumber on your eyelids to soothe the eyes and restore moisture.

Sink floaters

These simple ways to improve and maintain good vision can also help get rid of those annoying floaters in your eyes.

1) Roll your eyes in circles, starting at the top and slowly circling 10 times clockwise and 10 times counterclockwise.

2) Hold a pen at arm's length, focus your eyes on it, and slowly bring the pen closer until it's about six inches away from your nose. Then slowly move it back, keeping your eyes focused on the pen, 10 times in all.

3) Using your thumb knuckles, massage your temples in small circles, 20 times in one direction and 20 in the other.

4) With your thumb and index finger, pinch the area between your eyes, just above the bridge of the nose, and with the other hand gently massage the spot where the back of the head meets the neck. Pinch and massage at the same time; then switch hands and repeat.

After a month you will notice an improvement in vision and a decrease in floaters.

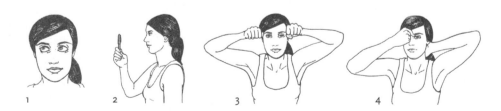

1   2   3   4

Juice up
your eyesight

An old Chinese folk remedy for cooling the liver and clearing the eyes is to drink a juice blend of celery, peppermint, and cilantro, made fresh daily. Thanks to modern research, we now know it's the *luteolin*, a bioflavonoid found in many herbs and in foods such as celery, basil, parsley, and peppermint. The subject of numerous animal and human studies, luteolin has been found to provide the best protection of cell DNA from radiation. There is some evidence that it helps protect the eye from UV radiation damage and from *glycation*, a process in which sticky sugar molecules bind up protein, potentially damaging the retina. Luteolin also acts as an antioxidant, promotes healthy blood sugar levels, and regulates insulin sensitivity. The typical dosage in supplement form is 200 mg a day, but I still favor the age-old Chinese beverage. Gear up your juicer!

Eat colorful foods
to prevent cataracts

A degenerative disorder of the eye characterized by cloudiness and darkened vision, *cataracts* usually show up as we get older, and the risk certainly rises after menopause. Certain conditions increase the chance of cataracts, including diabetes, trauma to the eyes, and hereditary defects. In the West, the common cure for cataracts is to have surgery. Don't let it go that far! Of course, if you already have severe cataracts that impair your vision, surgery may be your only recourse. But to prevent them or to treat mild, beginning-stage cataracts, choose natural methods. Cataracts form due to mineral imbalance within the lens of the eye, usually a result of free radical damage. That's why antioxidants in your diet are so important: Eat lots of fruits and vegetables, and be sure you get all colors of them every day. Go for foods rich in vitamin E (spinach), vitamin C (lemons), and beta-carotene (carrots). UV rays and nicotine both up the risk of cataracts. Wear sunglasses, and quit smoking cigarettes.

Natural supplements
keep cataracts at bay

If your vision is getting cloudy and you're already eating a diet high in colorful, antioxidant-rich food, it may be time to turn to natural supplements. Research points to a molecule called *pantethine*, which is present in all cells of the body, as a major actor in preventing the clumping of proteins in the eye. Pantethine is actually the active form of pantothenic acid, one of the B-complex vitamins. Other vitamins in the B family include inositol, which has also shown protective value against the onset of cataracts. In studies, high doses of vitamins E and C worked to prevent cataracts even in high-risk groups. I often recommend daily supplements of B vitamins including 800 mg of pantothenic acid, as well as E, C, beta-carotene, and selenium as your basic defense against cataracts.

CHAPTER 5

Energize Love and Sexuality

LOVE IS A POWERFUL FORCE expressed in many different ways, from romantic love to maternal love to universal spiritual love. To harness the energy of love in your Second Spring, as your life situation evolves, you want to reclaim your personal and sexual identity. Perimenopause and menopause are opportunities for a resurgence of libidinal pleasure; in postmenopause a woman can transform love and sexuality into experiences that are even more profound and fulfilling.

Romantic love is a double-edged sword, sustaining those who are happily attached to a mate but potentially devastating those who lose one. Maternal love is nurturing and even exhilarating in the attachment you feel for your child. Universal love and compassion free you from the anguish of loss and desire, and centers you in your essential oneness with every animate and inanimate thing.

Romantic Love: Fire and Water

Passionate love draws people together and opens the doorway to family-building, the cornerstone of human society. Interestingly, research shows that romantic love uses the same brain circuits as states of hunger, thirst, obsession, mania, and intoxication. It is no wonder that the behavior of people newly in love is sometimes likened to drunkenness! The love circuits trigger the sex center in the brain, which causes various hormones and neurochemicals to be released, including estrogen, testosterone, dopamine, and oxytocin; this in turn triggers the sexual impulse, pleasure, and lubrication. During this phase, your rational judgment is out the window, and the highs and lows of intense emotions virtually enslave you.

After the first year of being in love, or the "honeymoon" phase, the hunger-obsession-addiction chemicals are dialed down and replaced by the bonding and attachment circuits, which favor long-term pairing. This shift from manic love and sexuality to a calmer, attachment-oriented love is necessary to ensure the survival of the family—it is not a sign that love's flame has gone cold. Many married couples lament a loss of passion with their mate, yet take comfort in the stable, predictable nature of the relationship. Midlife may hold some pleasant surprises for them, as you will see in this chapter.

In Chinese medicine, the dynamics of emotional love and sexuality are expressed in the energies of the heart and kidney networks. The heart network correlates with the fire element and is the seat of emotional love; the kidney network, correlating with the water element, forms the foundation of sexual energy. The two elemental energies harmonize and converge, creating a natural union of love and sexual arousal. When the two energies decouple or are in disharmony due to emotional or health disturbances, sexual problems may arise. For most menopausal women, kidney energy becomes depleted, leading to a decline in hormonal secretion by the sex glands, and must be replenished for health and sexual fulfillment.

To counteract these changes, I recommend techniques that Chinese women have used for centuries: libido-enhancing food recipes, specific herbal formulas, and acupuncture. An active sex life is good for both your health and your relationship. The advice in this chapter can help you rekindle some of your buried passion.

Mature Love and the Uninhibited Libido

The love and bond cultivated between a couple over the years are strengthened by raising a family, living together with affection, and respecting and supporting one another. Your expressions of love for each other may change with time; happily married couples constantly explore various ways to manifest their love and stay attuned to their partners' needs. You naturally divide yourself between maternal love for your children and romantic love for your mate, but as you approach midlife and your children become more independent, you are free to devote more love to your mate. During your fertile years, even though your biology drives you to mate and bear children, your social brain restrains these impulses for practical socioeconomic reasons. Fear of pregnancy can inhibit libido, as can contraceptive methods and the stresses of a busy life. Some women find that their sex drive skyrockets during menopause, freed of such fears and stress. There are natural ways to unblock your sexual energy, restoring the union of fire and water energies, which I'll reveal in this chapter.

The Taoist tradition has long recognized the power of sexuality in health, longevity, and spirituality. Appropriateness and naturalness are the hallmarks of healthy sexuality. The three principles of a healthy sexuality are awareness, attunement, and consideration. The first principle means that you should be aware of your needs and make sure to communicate them. Do not force the act if it does not feel natural, if your energy is low, or if conditions are not safe and conducive. The second principle is to be in tune: Follow the seasons and observe that in nature animals tend to be more sexually active during spring and summer and less so during autumn and winter. Frequency of sex also depends on your health. The third principle calls for you to be considerate. It is equally important to gauge your partner's mood, energy, and needs so that you can respect and accommodate them. Achieving satisfaction for both partners is the first step toward reaping the benefits of sexuality.

The Power of the Feminine—Love and Compassion

Women more than men understand the healing power of love, which can break through blockages, overcome separation, ease pain, and comfort loss. Love is the power that unites humanity with the rest of the universe. A woman is naturally more spiritual. Feminine energy seeks to express itself as love and compassion for individuals as well as for all children and manifestations of the universal divine. By the time her own children are independent or nearly so, a woman can turn her loving capacity outward, into the world around her.

You can now use the wisdom and skills acquired through life experience to help your community while reinventing yourself. Many women go back to school, start new business endeavors, make new friends. Contributing to society and becoming a mentor to younger women is a way to pass on wisdom, once a natural tradition from mothers to daughters, grandmothers to granddaughters. In modern industrialized society, that has all but vanished from the domestic sphere, replaced by schools and workplaces. Yet you can share your wealth and knowledge in many ways, and you will be surprised at the intensity of the joy it brings you.

You will find satisfaction and purpose in your life in a loving, sexual relationship with your partner, your maternal love toward your offspring, and universal love and compassion for your neighbors, friends, co-workers, and even strangers. All these experiences are possible in your Second Spring. Here are some Chinese medicine secrets for achieving them.

Menopausal brain: new freedom, new behavior

During menopause your brain is rewired. The hormones active during the reproductive years are now no longer the main driver. It is often a time of self-discovery, when women decide to confront problems they were aware of in the past but too overburdened to address. Perhaps you've become much more passionate about correcting social and environmental injustices and have begun to devote yourself to acting on these issues. If you suppressed your ambitions for higher education or a career during the childbearing years, you can now act on your new-found freedom and energy—some women venture into new businesses, change careers, or go back to school.

Women in their Second Spring also commonly experience a stronger libido. This sexual energy can drive a zest to rearrange your life. Changes in the brain spur changes in behavior: Some women demand that their relationships change and evolve; some decide to leave unsatisfying situations. You can learn to harness this energy and make it work to your advantage.

Healthy loving
lengthens your life span

Healthy sex, nature's fountain of youth, raises your levels of endorphins, DHEA, and growth hormone, which increase longevity. Simultaneously, sex lowers levels of the stress hormones adrenaline and cortisol, which decrease your life span. While healthy loving adds years to your life, it also takes years off your face, making you actually *look* younger. Studies show that people who are highly satisfied with their sex life—meaning both its quantity and quality—looked 4 to 7 years younger than their peers. This results from reduced stress, greater happiness and contentment, and better sleep—in addition to the hormonal and chemical changes that satisfying sex can bring. So before you invest in a costly makeover, try improving your sex life.

Love stokes
the fire of sex

In traditional Chinese medicine, sexual health is the
function of the *yang*, or fire energy, of the kidney-adrenal
network. Yang energy may wane due to unhealthy dietary
or lifestyle factors, or become blocked by negative emotions.
When this happens, there is a deficiency of the fire that
sustains healthy sexual energy. To restoke these flames,
however, one must first understand how this fire energy
is lit. The heart network houses the spirit, which provides
the emotional connection that initially stokes the fire of
sexual arousal. In other words, love is the best aphrodisiac!
The spirit must be in harmony with fire energy, the basis
for physical attraction. For most women, reconnecting
with their own emotions, bonding with their partner, and
feeling desirable are essential to restoring libido. And for
the majority of men, physical fitness and relaxation can
increase sexual function and bolster confidence. For ultimate
sexual fulfillment, you must start by working on the love
between you and your partner. Try open communication,
let yourself be vulnerable, and love your partner for who
he is and not who you want him to be.

Food for sex

If you have the blahs in the sex department, it may be because of a nutritional deficiency. Instead of buying some new lingerie, try modifying your diet to include foods that have well-established benefits for the libido. Pungent, spicy foods—garlic, onions, chives, cinnamon, ginger, peppers, coriander, and cardamom—can activate arousal centers and increase blood flow to the lower body. Eating arginine-rich foods will keep you stoked with this amino acid, a precursor to the hormones testosterone and estrogen, so have plenty of eggs and meat in addition to the powerhouse sources, nuts and seeds. Shellfish such as oysters, clams, mussels, shrimp, and scallops contain a rich supply of zinc, which is also essential for manufacturing hormones. Eat right and you'll say *mm-mmm* in more ways than one!

Little miracle
from wild oats

The common oat plant, *Avena sativa*, has long been considered a sexual tonic. Besides its role as a healthy staple that lowers cholesterol and benefits the heart, oat contains a nutrient called *avenacoside*. This substance supports healthy testosterone levels by freeing bound-up, inaccessible testosterone and making it available to the system. The percentage of testosterone that is inaccessible rises with age. Why should midlife women care? A healthy testosterone level promotes libido in women as well as men, and increases muscle strength, energy endurance, and mental capacity.

Flax for your
flagging sex life

An ancient crop cultivated by the ancient Babylonians, *flaxseed*, also known as *linseed*, contains rich supply of lignans in its hull. Lignans are phytoestrogens that improve levels of good estrogens such as *estradiol*, which protects women from heart disease, bone loss, and vaginal dryness. It is also helpful in maintaining a healthy ratio of testosterone to its bound cousin, DHT. Optimal testosterone levels are essential to a peppy sex drive for women, as well as men. Studies have also found lignans to be beneficial during menopause as agents that prevent hair loss and acne, keep cholesterol and blood sugar in balance, and act as potent antioxidants. Flax oil contains only small amounts of lignan, so it is better to grind your own flaxseed, hulls and all. Try taking one tablespoon daily sprinkled over your breakfast grains or mixed in fruit juice or a smoothie.

Don't let your sedge
wither from the lake

In his famous poem "La Belle Dame Sans Merci," John Keats described the pain of lost love in the line: *"Though the sedge has withered from the lake, and no birds sing...."* Perhaps he knew that a plant belonging to the sedge family was a traditional herb for relieving pain and heightening sexual potency. The plant, *nutgrass* or *cyperus*, is used in Chinese medicine to treat liver energy blockage, which often leads to depression, menstrual pain, and indigestion. Japanese studies show that nutgrass extract has anti-coagulant properties, preventing platelets from clumping together to form clots. Additionally, it is used as a diuretic to treat high blood pressure. A recent Egyptian study of cyperus confirmed its value as a remedy for menstrual disorders thanks to its estrogen-balancing activity. Nutgrass can be taken as a tea, two to three cups a day, or as an herbal extract, typically up to 300 mg daily. It is available from health food stores, online, and from acupuncturists and herbalists.

Puncture vines spike up sexual energy

Within the arsenal of Chinese herbal libido tonics, *Tribulus terrestris* stands out as one of the most popular for improving sexual functions. Also known as *puncture vine*, it grows naturally throughout Asia, the Middle East, Europe, and the Americas and contains seeds that are sharp and painful to step on. Traditionally used in Chinese herbal formulas for liver, kidney, and cardiovascular conditions, tribulus has been found in animal studies to enhance testosterone release and increase endurance and strength. Additionally, some research has found tribulus to have antimicrobial and antitumor potential, and the saponin in the herb has anti-oxidant activity. Other benefits of tribulus include lowering blood pressure, cholesterol, and blood sugar. I recommend that my patients take 300 mg daily as a sexual tonic (men can take it too). It is available in health food stores, online, or from acupuncturists.

Libidinal lift
with sea cucumber

Growing up in Asia, when I attended lavish banquets and feasts I couldn't help noticing that women would rave about dishes of sea cucumber, which they declared, kept them youthful and even turned back the clock. This prized food fetches high prices in Asia for its anti-aging properties. Although it does come from the sea, it is not a cucumber but a marine animal related to sea urchins and starfish. It contains a rich supply of mucopolysaccharides and chondroitins—both excellent support for bones and joints—as well as vitamin A; thiamine, riboflavin, niacin, and other B vitamins; and minerals like calcium, iron, magnesium, and zinc. Maybe it's the high zinc content that makes sea cucumber so good for the libido and reproductive functions, as confirmed by modern studies. Those women were right: anti-aging and pro-libido . . . not a bad deal!

Nutty boost
for your libido

Everywhere in the world, especially throughout China
and the Middle East, people eat nuts and seeds for their
wonderful flavor, texture, and health-promoting properties.
Traditional Chinese herbal therapy prescribes nuts like
walnuts, almonds, and chestnuts along with sesame and
hemp seed as tonics for kidney vitality and sexual vigor.
With good reason! Modern studies show that nuts and
seeds are rich in the amino acid arginine, which appears
to restore declining levels of growth hormone to a range
typical of the prime years, thereby boosting sexual and
mental functions. Moreover, arginine is a precursor to the
neurotransmitter nitric oxide, important for normal blood
flow and pressure, healthy blood vessels, and proper
immune function. To give a boost to your sex life, you can
try taking 6 to 10 grams of arginine daily in supplement
form, but you may prefer to enjoy a handful of mixed nuts
and seeds for a snack every day—as I do.

Morinda:
berry sexy!

Commonly known by the commercial name *noni*, *morinda*
is a type of mulberry that has been used as an herbal remedy
throughout much of Asia and in Pacific Island societies.
While the commercial supplement is derived mostly from
the fruit, Chinese medicine has long used the more potent
morinda root as a longevity and sex tonic. The root is
traditionally prescribed for a wide range of problems, from
low libido in women to impotence in men as well as high
blood pressure, weak digestion, respiratory problems, and
immune dysfunction conditions. The herb also has been
found to increase energy and boost stamina and endurance. Morinda contains potassium, vitamin C, carotene,
vitamin A, flavonoids, linoleic acid, rutin, and other
phytonutrients. Often found with other herbs in libido-
and performance-enhancing formulations for both women
and men, it is available in health food stores, online, and
from acupuncturists and Chinese herbalists.

When your love life is history, update it with histidine

Found in abundance in poultry, saltwater fish, meat, eggs, and soy, histidine is a semiessential amino acid that helps your body digest protein, protect red blood cells, and maintain healthy immune function. However, histidine's major claim to fame is that it can help increase sexual arousal. Women who take histidine an hour before sexual activity experienced enhanced arousal and intensified feeling. The same amino acid may benefit older men's sexual performance as well. Other benefits of histidine include suppressing an overactive appetite and assisting the body in the removal of accumulated heavy metals. As a supplement, typical dosage is around 500 mg a day, but whenever possible, go for the natural sources in food.

Horny goat weed:
the name says it all

Thousand of years ago, Chinese shepherds observed that goats, after eating certain weeds, would become sexually energized and active. The same weed was used as a traditional remedy for disorders of the kidneys, joints, adrenal glands, and liver. Lo and behold, patients got well, but that wasn't all they got! Soon Chinese doctors began prescribing it to increase libido and sexual function. Nowadays, it is believed to promote blood flow to the reproductive organs and possibly mimic the effects of sex hormones. Horny goat weed stimulates the sensory nerves and increases sexual desire in both men and women by supporting essential neurotransmitters that play a role in sexual arousal. It also counters fatigue and is considered a longevity herb. To show results, it is typically taken daily. The herb is available in health food stores, online, and from Asian pharmacies and acupuncturists, often in a formula with other natural libido-boosters.

Cardamom:
bees do it!

In Asia, cardamom has long been valued medicinally for its ability to increase circulation and improve energy. Used routinely as a spice in cooking, especially poultry and red meat dishes, cardamom also gives chai tea its main flavor. Cardamom is a stimulant with a positive effect on overall well-being, both as a tonic for the body and as an anti-depressant for emotional disorders. Orchid bees are drawn to cardamom as well, and use it to synthesize pheromones. Thanks to this combination of properties, cardamom is often prescribed by Chinese doctors, in doses up to 5 grams daily, to revitalize sexual desire. In addition, the spice is an antacid, reduces fever, and eases indigestion. It also combats intolerance to grains, so add some to your breakfast cereal or bake it into breads and cakes for a delicious taste and untroubled digestion.

Peppery daikon
puts pep in your loving

With a long history in Asia as an excellent therapeutic food, daikon radish is traditionally used to activate the respiratory system, expel mucus, and serve as a mild diuretic. It has also been shown to aid in the metabolism of fat and it may help ward off cancer. But the versatile vegetable has another interesting property: Daikon is highly beneficial for sexual function, stimulating a waning libido in both men and women and even promoting fertility. The seed is particularly effective; buy it from health food stores in tea form and drink two cups a day. If you prefer, you can eat daikon in soup or salad just like any other radish. With a difference!

Snake's nest seed:
libido-enhancing secret

Ancient legend has it that a Chinese prince, desperately in love with a wife who suffered from frigidity, sought the advice of an old farmer who had 18 children. The man told him to look for an herb that grew around snake burrows and give her the fruit to eat, and her problem would soon disappear. That is how cnidium got its common name, *snake's nest seed*—and the prince and the princess lived happily ever after. Since then, this Chinese herb has traditionally been used to increase sexual desire and function in both men and women. Studies have found a natural phytochemical in cnidium called *osthol* that may help increase the level of sex hormones and promote blood flow to the genitals. Some of my female patients have attested to its libido-enhancing qualities. Side benefits of cnidium, according to animal studies, include the potential to prevent osteoporosis and asthma. I recommend my patients take 100 to 200 mg about an hour before sexual activity, or on a daily basis to restore normal libidinal energy. It is available in health food stores, online, and from acupuncturists and Chinese herbalists.

A rose is arouse is a rose

The Crusaders returned home with rose plants, which were then cultivated by monks for their therapeutic properties. The discovery of *Rosa chinensis* in China at the end of the 18th century gave birth to the modern garden rose. Today, the rose is almost universally associated with love and happiness. In Chinese tradition, a rose is traditionally put into rice wine to stimulate loving relationships, as the rose's essential oil may be a medicinal boost for the libido. Herbalists use this symbol of love as an antidote for sadness and hangovers; Bach flower remedies include the rose to cure apathy. Its essential oil also helps regulate menstruation, soothe PMS, and diminish postpartum depression. Rosehips, rich in vitamin C, promote healing and immune functions. Rose petal tea soothes the emotions and helps eliminate toxins by cleansing the liver and gall bladder; the petals can also be added to black or green tea to soften the bitterness of the tannin.

Down-home aphrodisiac: the smell of pumpkin pie

When you arrange your home to please the senses, you tend to think of colors you like, objects and pictures that bring you enjoyment, even sounds that create a harmonious atmosphere. You may even pay attention to scent, usually floral bouquets, or perhaps a lemony room freshener. But how about delightful cooking smells? There is nothing like certain familiar odors wafting through the house to make you smile. A few good examples are chocolate chip cookies, baked apples, and pumpkin pie. Now here's an unusual tip: You can use that mm-mm cooking smell to perk up your sex life. Studies have found that certain smells can increase blood flow to the penis and excite a man sexually. They include pumpkin pie, black licorice, and vanilla. Do I hear you turning the pages of your cookbook?

Make time
for intimacy

If making love is important to you, put it on the calendar. You may cringe at first—an appointment to have sex? We like to think of lovemaking as a spontaneous act, but it is also something we need to put a little energy into. In any case, after being married for 10, 15, 20 years or longer, spontaneity may be difficult to act on. By planning you give your time together more attention. Perhaps you make a special dinner, set the table in a more romantic way, prepare a bath ahead of time. Looking forward to your date can spice up your mood—your mate's, too—in anticipation. Planning can revitalize your sex life and marriage.

Restore natural lubrication and vaginal health

Vaginal dryness, one of the symptoms of menopause and hormonal imbalance, can make intercourse painful and sometimes even lead to bleeding—a big deterrent to your sex life! Instances of bacterial and yeast infections may also rise. As you revitalize your overall well-being with the tips in this book, your natural lubrication will improve. In the meantime, you can use aloe vera with vitamin E gel as an effective lubricant that is completely chemical-free.

In Chinese medicine, we help women restore a natural, healthy vaginal environment with vaginal probiotics—both as pills taken orally and as suppositories that dissolve in the vaginal canal—or simply with plain organic yogurt used as a cream. This will lubricate and soothe the tissues as well as restore the natural flora.

Additionally, because these problems are due to decreased estrogen output, I suggest applying phyto-estrogen cream, which contains the natural plant-based hormone, for topical relief. Consistent use can restore the lubrication, tone, and plumpness of the vagina with little risk of side effects or complications. Lastly, be sure to do your kegel exercises—they're simple: just tighten and release your vaginal muscles 10 times—to increase blood flow in the area.

Strengthen your bladder
with lotus seed

The seed of the lotus blossom is a powerful herb in Chinese medicine, and one that comes in handy for a woman at this stage of life. The hormonal change you are going through can cause unexpected side effects such as leaking urine when you laugh too hard. Lotus seed boosts kidney function, alkalizes the blood, and strengthens the bladder, improving urinary function. There are several ways to incorporate lotus seed into your diet. You can buy the dried seeds from an Asian market, soak them overnight, and then use them in soups or dishes with beans or lentils. The crystallized seeds can be consumed as a snack, and lotus paste makes a sweet addition to baked goods. Lotus seed extract, another convenient way to use this gift from nature, is available at Asian pharmacies or online.

Cinnamon combats
bladder infections

In the United States, cinnamon is usually thought of as the delicious spice in a breakfast roll or apple pie filling. But in other parts of the world, especially India and Asia, cinnamon is a healing herb. Among other medicinal uses, it acts to purify the blood, detoxify the system, improve the digestion of fats, stimulate brain function, and regulate blood sugar in patients with type 2 diabetes. Most significant for women are its antiseptic properties and its ability to fight bladder infection. As hormonal changes progress during midlife, the immune system of the urinary tract can grow weaker, leading to more frequent infections. The remedy I recommend is to take 5,000 milligrams of vitamin C every two or three hours with a cup of strong cinnamon tea. If the infection remains for more 48 hours, you need to call your doctor. Cinnamon tea can also help promote menstruation and allay menstrual pain.

Cranberry: an infection fighter to be thankful for

Perimenopause usually brings with it a decline in the immune resistance of the mucus membranes lining the vagina, cervix, bladder wall, and urethra, making both vaginal and urinary tract infections more common. Today, drinking cranberry juice is widely used to prevent bladder infection. The berry contains a substance that keeps bacteria from adhering to the bladder wall, causing them to be washed out with the stream of urine. Cranberry juice is believed to be most effective when drunk regularly, which appears to reduce the frequency of recurrent bladder infections in women prone to develop them. If a bladder infection does occur, drinking cranberry juice may help you heal, along with high doses of vitamin C and plenty of water. Drink a little of the juice daily for prevention, or try taking 300 to 400 mg in capsule form twice daily to treat an infection.

Reverse prolapse without surgery

Among the aging effects women experience is a weakening of the pelvic tissue that holds organs in place, causing them to hang low, or prolapse. *Uterine prolapse* is most common, but it can happen to the bladder and stomach as well. About one in every four women over 60 suffers prolapse, which can result in pain, frequent urination or incontinence, swelling in the abdomen, and discomfort during intercourse. Western medicine offers surgery to lift the drooping organs, but you can prevent and even reverse prolapse with a yoga pose. Perform the Shoulder Stand twice a day for five minutes: Lie down on your back and, using both arms to support your lower back, raise your feet, legs, hips, and back to a vertical position, so your upper back and shoulders are holding you up. You may use the wall to support you at first, but try to gradually strengthen your pelvic muscles until you can do the pose unassisted. As an added benefit, you are driving blood flow to your brain. That's smart!

CHAPTER 6

Lift Your Mood
Promote Restorative Sleep

THE RICHNESS OF YOUR FEMININE EMOTIONS is a treasure to be cherished. Your ability to experience and express deep emotions allows you to connect with people on a profound level and feel empathy and compassion. Women generally are better than men at expressing their inner reality, coping with stressful life situations, and maintaining community. Being in touch with your emotions has other benefits: Women live longer than men due to their lower rates of stress-induced illness. Maternal love makes women the keepers of the family flame. Studies show that in primitive cultures, families whose grandmothers aided in foraging and cared for their grandchildren were more likely to survive and pass on the family lineage. Women's particular emotional qualities, which begin to emerge as early as 2 years of age, are necessary for the survival and health of the human race.

Emotions have two sides: bright and dark, pleasant and upsetting, healthy and unhealthy. You have some choice in which side to be on. Choosing to be on the bright side does not mean that you never feel pain, but when a situation pulls you into sadness, you will not dwell there for long. When you accept that conflicts are inevitable, you realize that resolving them is part of your life—and in the end, this helps you grow and makes you stronger.

Emotional Challenges at Midlife

In midlife, however, unpredictable and surprising emotional changes can occur. Some of the causes are physiological, driven by hormones, and others psychological, resulting from unhappiness with life's circumstances. The resulting mood swings, from sudden bursts of anger to depression to panic attacks, can become unbearable. Thirty percent of women in perimenopause and menopause are relatively symptom-free, but many perimenopausal women experience continuous premenstrual syndrome (PMS) for 10 to 15 years before menopause, with symptoms of depression, anxiety, irritability, restless sleep, weight gain, and food cravings.

In Chinese medicine, mood and sleep disorders in women have roots in the heart and the liver. The organ network housing the spirit is the heart. With all her attention focused on family members, work, and other priorities, a woman's spirit becomes troubled, and she lies awake at night with an aching, unfulfilled heart. The liver network, when healthy, ensures emotional spontaneity and acts as a pressure valve to release emotions when they are suppressed, as they often are for women in our society. A blockage of liver energy manifests as depression, anxiety, and other mood disorders. Because the female body is wise, it produces these emotional and physical symptoms as a form of feedback—messages that you need to attend to your own personal and emotional needs. If you acknowledge your feelings, take time to nurture your spirit, and fulfill the best impulses of your heart, your body will gradually return to normal.

The Mood Cocktail: Genetics, Hormones, Stress

The escalation in PMS symptoms reflects several factors: genetic makeup, shifting hormone levels, and stress. Genetics play a role in menstrual and pregnancy patterns, which often closely mirror those of your mother and grandmother. If your mother experienced PMS and early menopause, you are likely to experience the same and start yours early, too.

As your estrogen starts to drop and follicle-stimulating hormones rise after your mid-thirties, neurotransmitters like serotonin, dopamine, and norepinephrine also begin to fluctuate wildly, contributing to mood swings and sleep problems. Your nervous system goes into overdrive, putting you in an almost constant fight-or-flight state. The key to restoring balance to the system is to support the nerve functions that produce and release neurochemicals like *dopamine* and *oxytocin*, which are responsible for states of bliss and tranquillity. Exercise, meditation, acupuncture, and herbal therapy are some natural ways to address hormonal imbalance and lift mood. Acupuncture especially has been shown to be effective in improving levels of serotonin and other calming neurotransmitters.

Stress is often overlooked as a factor in midlife mood swings. Many women in our society perform like superwomen, holding down full-time jobs while shouldering primary responsibility for child care and household management. If they have elderly or ailing parents, they often take care of them, too. They may be obligated to assume these duties, but sometimes it is their personality that drives these superwomen to take on all tasks and strive for perfection in everything they do. Their high expectations of themselves and others cause frustrations for them and for those around them.

Even if you aren't a perfectionist, at this stage of life you may find that demands on you just continue to escalate, with no relief in sight. Disagreements and conflicts may become more frequent; resentments in relationships can boil over with increasing vehemence. No wonder many women find themselves depressed, angry, sleepless, and spent. Depleted emotionally and physically, they are highly vulnerable to sleep and mood disorders.

Use East and West Together

Sleep and mood disorders share many common traits. Physiologically both involve low levels of serotonin in the brain and thus react adversely to *cortisol*, the stress hormone your body produces under conditions of prolonged stress and tension. Typical treatments in Western medicine involve drug therapy with antidepressants that are selective serotonin reuptake inhibitor (SSRIs) along with sleeping pills, which can both be helpful for cases of serious clinical depression. If you are reluctant to use drug therapy due to its side effects and addictive nature, however, a number of natural remedies using herbs, nutritional supplements, and meditation practices are available. Would you like to sleep like a baby without taking drugs? Try meditation—especially the **Stress Release Meditation** on page 220—it works for the majority of my insomniac patients.

Mood disorders like depression can involve a range of emotions that you may need to acknowledge. Various psychotherapeutic approaches address the emotional spectrum of depression quite effectively, especially cognitive therapy. Acupuncture helps to stimulate the body's physiological production and balance of neurochemicals, so it is often used as a complementary treatment to conventional psychopharma-cology and psychotherapy. Work with your doctors to find the best solution for your mood and sleep problems.

Your Second Spring is a time of empowerment and release, so I hope you will take advantage of the many tips in this chapter that can help you maintain or regain a stable emotional footing.

Daily rituals
keep you centered

When you have symptoms of menopause, it means that your body is essentially trying to make more estrogen. The pituitary gland in the brain, sensing a lack of the hormone, attempts to stimulate the ovaries to produce more. Estrogen levels fluctuate drastically in response, resulting in hot flashes, emotional swings, and agitation. To counteract the chaotic adjustment going on in your body, establish a series of rituals that will stabilize your system.

1) Choose a particular time during daylight hours to engage in exercise. This will rebalance your chemistry.

2) One hour before bedtime, reprogram your brain by dimming the lights. This helps the brain and body prepare to sleep.

3) Take a bath in Epsom salts, scent the air with lavender, and write in a journal to get thoughts out of your mind and down on paper. This will help your mind and body calm down.

4) In the morning, start the day with meditation. Spend 10 to 15 minutes in meditative relaxation, with calming music if you desire.

Replace negative
with positive thoughts

Recent studies show that a typical woman has 60,000 thoughts a day, 80 percent of them negative. Imagine what this is doing to your body! In the West, people often have to be reminded that there is a synergy between mind and body; in Chinese science, they have never been split apart. The body reacts to your thoughts just as it reacts to things like light, temperature, and nutrition. You can feed your body with healthy, nourishing mental energy by reframing the way you say things to yourself. Instead of letting your thoughts run wild with anxiety, fear of failure, or resentment, say to yourself, "I am proactive. I am diligent. I can handle the tasks I have ahead of me. I have just the right amount of work. I enjoy my responsibilities and fulfill them well." In fact, repeating positive affirmations can actually suppress the cortisol that the adrenal gland releases in times of stress—decreasing your stress level and leaving you peaceful and calm.

Change
bad attitudes

I have heard people acknowledge that some part of their personality is a deterrent to achieving what they want—whether health, happiness, or personal fulfillment—yet they believe they can do nothing about it. This attitude is self-defeating. We all have the power to change, no matter how ingrained our particular personality traits. Two of them are particularly harmful.

First is the tendency toward hostility and anger: You are easily upset, fly off the handle, take offense quickly. Studies show that people with hostile personalities are four to five times more likely to die between the ages of 25 and 50 than their nonhostile counterparts.

The second dangerous trait is negativity and moroseness. You don't necessarily suffer from clinical depression, but you focus on the downside of things. If so, your immune function may be weak, making you more vulnerable to cancer and heart disease, research indicates.

Recognize yourself? That's the first step. Cognitive therapy can help you become more aware and change your behavior. Meditation practice is another path that changes your brain for the better. Studies show that people who meditate are calmer, slower to anger, and better able to see past problems to good outcomes. Start now. There's no better time to change than during the change.

A sunny mood—
not just a metaphor

If you are feeling blue, whatever the reason, simply taking
a walk outside on a sunny day can give you a lift. Studies
show that exposure to sunlight stimulates the *pineal
gland*, a small organ located behind your forehead that
produces a hormone called *melatonin*. Melatonin helps
keep our body clock on time, regulating the circadian
rhythm that controls appetite, sleep, and sex hormones.
The pineal gland also affects the production of other brain
chemicals such as *serotonin*, the neurotransmitter sometimes called the mood chemical. By getting sufficient sunlight throughout the seasons, you can improve your mood
and prevent *seasonal affective disorder* (SAD), a form
of depression common in northern areas of the globe that
get little sunlight during the winter months. If you live
in these regions or are especially susceptible to SAD,
I recommend using full-spectrum lightbulbs, which have
been shown to diminish the effects of SAD and elevate
your mood naturally.

The color of calm: blue

Try this experiment: Ask all your friends to name their favorite color. It's a good bet the vast majority will choose blue, the perennial favorite. Studies show that people who love blue tend to be even-tempered, cool, and no-nonsense. But even if it isn't your own top choice, that doesn't mean you don't need a dose of blue from time to time. Blue is the perfect color for relaxation, because it actually stimulates the brain to produce calming hormones like serotonin and dopamine. If you need a change of mood or some relaxation after a particularly stressful day, just looking at a blue sky or staring into a pool of blue water can help soothe you. The color may even benefit sleep. Paint your bedroom hues of blue or bluish green and go there to meditate, rest, or read a book surrounded by this serene color.

In touch
heal for real

Nowadays we have so many options to connect with our loved ones—email, cell phones, personal Web sites, and snail mail—but do we feel connected? These methods all have their advantages, but as a woman you need something more. You need to connect with others on a physical level, through the eyes, through touching and being touched. If you find yourself spending most of your day alone, reach out. As often as you can, be in the physical presence of people you love. Babysit for your siblings or friends or take care of your own grandchildren, who often give loving hugs spontaneously. Join groups of people who share similar interests and gather together in person. Feel your presence in the world and make it felt by others.

Start your art— now's the time!

As the door of procreative capacity closes, another door of creativity opens. Step through it! Art is a powerful way to restore a sense of inner balance and bring joy and happiness to the heart. Find an art medium you have an affinity with and indulge yourself, even if you've never tried it before. Artistic activities like drawing or painting, projecting your feelings onto a canvas, let you acknowledge the emotions you are going through and free your spirit. Singing or playing a musical instrument help feelings emerge as sound and tone. Movement such as dance or mime is a wonderful way to explore and tap into your inner self through physical action. Knitting, needlework, scrapbooking, calligraphy, and photography are all creative, inspiring activities. I find flower arrangement a fun way to express myself, and some of my friends revel in pottery and cooking. Whatever you choose, art can help you plumb your own latent potential.

The perfect chemistry: GABA and your brain

Midlife involves so many stressors—job, family, your changing body—and all take a toll on your brain. A healthy brain has a balanced chemistry and can deal better with stress. Some neurotransmitters excite the nerves and others calm the nerves; one of these chemicals, GABA (gamma amino butyric acid), is especially helpful when tension strikes. As the primary neurotransmitter for calming nerve signals, it prevents stress- or anxiety-related messages from reaching the brain. Unfortunately, the body's production of the chemical wanes with time, and low levels of GABA can increase anxiety, insomnia, irritability, and depression. GABA has additional benefits for the aging body: It stimulates the pituitary gland to produce human growth hormone and may even help with weight loss. I suggest that my patients take 250 to 500 mg a day as a dietary supplement, along with vitamin B6, which helps your body use GABA.

Peony for
your thought

Flowers can help you deal with mood shifts and get you back in emotional balance. I'm not talking about aromatherapy or a bouquet from a loved one, but peony blossom, which is traditionally used to regulate menstruation, balance the hormonal system, and calm the emotions. In animal studies, peony extracts have been found to enhance mental function. The flower's abundant proanthocyanins and flavonoids are helpful antioxidants, as well. Peony is part of a traditional Chinese herbal formula called "Xiao Yao San" or simply "PMS," used for calming premenstrual symptoms. When taken with licorice root, the combination relieves muscle and menstrual cramps. The formula and peony blossoms alone are available in herb stores, online, and from acupuncturists and herbalists.

Rx for angst: pen and paper

Western medicine offers various ways to handle the emotional upheaval of perimenopause, sometimes with drugs or therapy. Yet one of the best ways to deal with your emotions is perhaps the simplest: Write down your feelings. Keeping a journal is a way to move energy, channel it, and ultimately release it. You don't have to do it forever, but try writing for at least 10 minutes a day (more if you feel like it) for at least a month or so. Give yourself time to spot some patterns in your emotions—and see if they correspond to any physical symptoms in your body. As you write, take the position of observer: Record your emotions without judging them; don't try to change or censor them. Let them out. Admit them to yourself. If you feel angry, don't try to correct it right now. Just write it down so that you can see clearly what is going on inside. Accept it, then work with it. You might be acknowledging these feelings for the first time after having swept them under the carpet. The next step is to identify the source of any anger, sadness, or other unhappiness so you can begin to make changes. Write in your journal every day, several times a day—you'll find it an excellent opportunity for transformation.

When emotions are stuck in your body

Many people store emotions in the body instead of releasing them via a healthy outlet and eventually experience physical pains as a result. Frequent symptoms that indicate you may have trapped feelings in your body are pains in the back, neck, shoulders, jaw area, or stomach. Sometimes it will be congestion in the ear or nose, the feeling of a lump stuck in your throat, chest tightness, or shortness of breath. Often we don't recognize the sensations that indicate we have pent-up, unexpressed emotions within our bodies, instead attributing the symptoms to other causes. But if you don't address these emotions, the blockages can cause even more serious harm to your health down the road—they can become chronic pain or even growths such as tumors and cancer. You need to free negative emotions by promoting energy flow within the body. Be alert to the symptoms when they arise, and use massage therapy, exercise, yoga, tai chi, or qi gong to get the circuits moving. By doing this now, you're preventing illness later in life.

Your liver: the heart of the emotions

In Chinese medicine, the liver is the seat of emotional expression. When you suppress your emotions it harms the liver. Conversely, if the liver is ailing, it will cause extreme outbursts of emotion or the opposite, an inability to express your emotions freely. How do we take care of the liver? The color that corresponds to the liver is green; in Chinese medicine, that means we need to eat green foods. Chlorophyll is a purifier and cleanser of the liver. In your daily diet, eat lots of green leafy vegetables, barley grass, seaweed, anything with chlorophyll. Be sure you exercise to keep the blood circulating and to release physical tension. Gentle movements promote smooth flow of energy and are always preferable to strenuous workouts that cause jarring, jagged energy patterns. Keep your liver healthy and it will pay off for your emotional health as well.

Berries, roots, and dandelion for a healthy liver

The liver is the body's ultimate multitasker. It detoxifies, aids in metabolism, stores energy, and secretes bile for digestion. In Chinese medicine, it is also seen to regulate emotional well-being. The best way to take care of your liver is by eating lots a green leafy vegetables and engaging in gentle exercise to keep it functioning at its peak. But if you do develop liver problems, or if you feel you need a little extra help, try the following herbs: Schisandra berry protects the liver from chemicals and calms the spirit. 200 mg daily for a month is the recommended dose for emotional anxiety. Dandelion will also clear and cleanse the liver and help release built-up anger. That dosage is 500 mg daily for a month or longer. Finally, white peony root is a Chinese herb traditionally used to soothe the liver and balance the mood. I recommend that my patients take 400 mg daily for one to three months. All the herbs are available from health food stores and Eastern medicine practitioners.

Best meds for heart palpitations: meditation

At midlife, some women suddenly wake up with frightening heart palpitations for the first time in their lives. In many cases this is due to the release of epinephrine during the change. Other times it may signal more serious heart problems, perhaps a latent mitral prolapse, coronary artery blockage, or a genetic or neurological condition. Go to your internist first for an EKG and treadmill stress test to rule out any serious heart problems. If nothing turns up, the palpitations may be part of perimenopause. Don't let the symptoms scare you. Instead, try meditation to help you gain control of them. If you awake each day with heart palpitations or fast pulse, start with a calming meditation. Meditate again before bedtime. When you're completely unwound before going to sleep, you'll wake up in better shape. In Chinese pharmacies, look for this traditional herbal formula: lily balm to calm the mind and nerves; senega root, a heart tonic that expels mucus and dampness; and the relaxing chamomile flower. Also, eliminate or cut back on caffeine—you may be more sensitive to it now, even if you could tolerate it when you were younger. Instead, switch to green tea or black tea. You'll be calmer, plus you'll reap the benefits of tea's antioxidant properties.

For good night's sleep, go easy on the alcohol

It's common for people to go to sleep without a problem after a few drinks, then wake up in the middle of the night. This unhealthy pattern disrupts the REM sleep you need and robs you of a good night's rest. Why does it happen? Alcohol is a depressant, so it makes you feel drowsy, and for the first four to five hours it may help relax you as you sleep. After that period the alcohol begins to wear off and your body undergoes a form of withdrawal, causing you to wake up. For an uninterrupted, restorative night of sleep, your best move is to stop drinking alcohol altogether. But if you are going to drink, make sure you do so early in the evening, preferably at dinner with your food. Having a cocktail before dinner is another option that won't interfere with your sleep.

Press here for a good night's sleep

Acupressure is a wonderful self-healing technique that anyone can perform. Here are two acupressure points you can use to help yourself go to sleep. One, called *Inner Gate*, or more technically *Pericardium-6*, is located near your wrist on your inner arm. To locate it, line up your index, middle, and ring fingers on the opposite arm so that your ring finger touches the crease on the inside of your wrist. The index finger is now touching P-6, a point between the two tendons on the inner arm. Mark it with a pen. Now use your thumb to press down on that point for 30 seconds, let go for five, and continue this sequence for five minutes, breathing deeply. Repeat on the other side. The second point, called *Kidney-1* or *Bubbling Spring*, is on the bottom of your foot, at the center of the indentation below the ball of your foot. Press down with your thumb, hold for 30 seconds, relax for five, and again continue for five minutes. There is no need to do both sides every night—just perform about 10 minutes of acupressure for a deep, calming sleep.

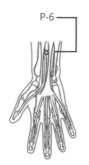

P-6

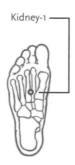

Kidney-1

Sleep tight with the dragon's eye on duty

With a taste and shape similar to lychee, *longan* or *dragon's eye fruit* has many therapeutic qualities. When premenopause has you on edge, longan calms your spirit and allays insomnia. It also nourishes the blood, promotes good vision, and strengthens the bladder to stop incontinence, another potential annoyance during the transition. Longan fruit contains substantial amounts of vitamins A and C, as well as minerals your body needs now: iron, magnesium, phosphorus, and potassium. Longan's use as a tonic herb in Chinese medicine may be due to its phenolic acids, which protect the liver and possess antioxidants. The dried fruit makes a wonderful snack to add to trail mix. You can find fresh and dried longan at Asian markets, in select health food stores, and online. Eat a small handful a day for peaceful sleep at night.

Powerful jujube against
insomnia and fatigue

In Chinese medicine, the heart is said to house the spirit. When the heart is weak, the spirit grows restless and cannot properly rest at night, so you experience insomnia or else sleep poorly and wake up unrefreshed. The herbal remedy for this condition is the seed of the jujube date. A traditional sedative, jujube seed calms the spirit, strengthens the heart, and facilitates good sleep. Research has shown the seed to be rich in saponins, which reduce irritability, anxiety, and fatigue while promoting relaxation and sleep. One big plus with jujube seed is that it doesn't make you tired when you take it during the daytime—in fact, it seems to promote clarity and reduce fatigue related to nervousness. Recommended dosage is up to 500 mg daily. You can find jujube seed in health food stores, online, and from acupuncturists and Chinese herbalists, usually combined in a formula with other natural herbs.

Passiflora for peaceful sleep

Passion flower, or passiflora, is a generous gift from nature found in various species throughout the world, and its medicinal properties are valued everywhere. Passion flower is a fruit that makes a delicious juice; its fresh or dried leaves are traditionally used as a therapeutic tea to treat insomnia, hot flashes, muscle spasms, and nervous digestive disorders. A recognized sedative found in many calm-inducing preparations, it contains harmala alkaloids, which prevent the breakdown of neurotransmitters like serotonin and dopamine, thus improving mood and promoting restful sleep. Passion flower is also known for its pain-relieving properties and may act to fight H. pylori, the bacteria that causes ulcers. To make a tea, steep 1 to 2 heaping tablespoons of the dried herb in one cup of hot water and drink just before bedtime. If you prefer the supplement form, the typical dosage is 200 mg at night.

Sweet dreams! The Chinese cure for insomnia

In Chinese medicine, we recognize that the female essence, or yin, slowly becomes depleted during menopause. Yin is a calming essence needed to balance the fiery yang, so when you are low on yin one major symptom is insomnia, manifested as difficulty falling asleep or episodes of waking up late at night and being unable to sleep again. Hot flashes, night sweats, irritability, and agitation are all related to this root condition. To ensure a good night's sleep, take a calming tea before bedtime. Look for one with the traditional Chinese herbs zizyphus seed, bamboo shavings, and oyster shell, which soothe the mind and spirit. Another natural sleep aid is the supplement 5-HTP, derived from an African plant, which converts to serotonin in the brain and has a tranquilizing effect. The typical dosage is 200 mg at night. Lastly, soaking your feet in a hot bath before you go to bed will produce a healthy relaxation response.

Deep exhalation
for deep sleep

Breathing is such an unconscious act that most of us only become aware of it when we need to gasp for air. That's why our focus tends to be on inhalation. But the secret to good breathing practices lies in exhalation, which expels toxins from your body and relaxes you. It's yin and yang at work: The inhale is a yang action; the exhale is yin, when everything deflates, loosens, moves out of you. Here's how to experience deep relaxation and improved sleep. When you inhale, fill up your abdomen first, watch it rise, then fill up your chest, so that the ribs expand. On exhale, let the air out of the ribs, then out of the abdomen, compressing your belly to make sure all the air is out. When you don't think you can exhale anymore, push out some more air, then more, until there is nothing left to expel. Now repeat the process slowly and deliberately. By the end of the fifth exhalation, you'll find yourself gloriously calm, even dreamy.

Overcome sleep apnea
before it overcomes you

Do you have trouble staying awake to get through your day? Do you feel sleepy all the time? Mentally foggy? You might be suffering from sleep apnea, a common condition that is often undiagnosed. People with sleep apnea stop breathing multiple times during the night and wake up gasping for air—or not at all. Sleep apnea causes nearly 40,000 deaths a year. Simple, natural solutions may help. First, if you are overweight, trim down. Excess fatty tissue in the back of the throat can obstruct the upper airway, causing you to stop breathing. Many people overcome apnea simply by losing weight. Second, always sleep on your side, never on your back. Third, don't get overtired. Take a little nap during the day, pace yourself to avoid overwork, and establish a regular sleep pattern. If none of this works, see your doctor and get a breathing device called a *CPAP* that delivers oxygen at night.

Three-scent
sleep remedy

After a stressful day, how do you wind down and clear your mind? Relaxing in a comfy chair, putting on some soothing sounds, and reading something light and entertaining are all good methods to get ready for some restful sleep. But as you ease your frazzled senses, don't forget your sense of smell. Certain aromas can fill you with feelings of tranquility, and research has found that lavender, vanilla, and green apple are among the best smells to help lower anxiety and induce sleep. You can use essential oils of these scents by applying them to the back of your neck or the inside of your wrist; even better, indulge in a warm bath with these oils dissolved in the water. Before bed, you might enjoy a glass of hot soy milk with natural vanilla flavoring for a calming effect inside and out.

Stop restless leg syndrome
with Epsom salts

It's annoying to sleep next to someone who has restless leg syndrome, and it's even worse if you have it. RLS disrupts your sleep and never allows you to reach the deep state you need in order to feel refreshed in the morning. When you have this condition, your nervous system sends random impulses to your legs at night, causing involuntary jerks and shudders. Of course, Western science offers medications for this, but why not avoid their potential side effects and take a drug-free approach? Try soaking your feet in a hot Epsom salts bath and massaging them. This calms the entire nervous system, especially your legs, as your body absorbs the magnesium sulfate that constitutes the salts. You can also try taking 500 mg of magnesium in supplement form before bedtime for a similar effect, calming the legs and promoting a good night's sleep.

CHAPTER 7

Increase Circulation
Cool the Flashes

YOU'RE SITTING ACROSS FROM YOUR FRIEND having a casual conversation and suddenly, without warning, a rush of heat covers your chest, throat, and face, accompanied by heart palpitations, skin redness, and beads of sweat dripping down your chest. You quickly take off your jacket, only to put it back on a few minutes later, just as suddenly feeling chilled. This episode is repeated anytime and anywhere, whether you are calm, anxious, excited, or depressed. What is happening? Welcome to hot flashes, the most common symptom of menopause, affecting some 80 percent of all women.

Yin, Yang, and Your Heart

Several circulatory conditions can affect women near midlife and beyond, including fast heartbeat, hot flashes, plaque in the arteries, and varicose veins. In Chinese medicine, good circulation is key to good health, and a large percentage of all illnesses are attributed to blocked flow of vital blood and energy to critical areas of the body. Blood delivers nutrients and oxygen to the tissues and transports waste products to be eliminated. When any part of the estimated 100,000 mile-long vascular network of arteries, veins, and capillaries in the human body becomes obstructed, a break in function may ensue, sometimes with grave consequences such as a stroke, blood clot, or heart attack. However, if you start now, natural approaches to circulation health can prevent these potential problems.

In Chinese medicine, estrogen and other hormones are considered yin, or the cooling, material aspect of the body, and are primarily associated with the kidney network. Hormonal decline, a drop in yin, causes the energy balance to shift toward yang, and thus elevated heat. The heart, extremely sensitive to heat energy, becomes restless, agitated, and irritable. Not coincidentally, Chinese medicine recommends cultivating love and compassion to counterbalance excess heat energy and calm the resulting disturbance of the spirit. A basic tenet of the Taoist science of longevity is that the human body is highly regenerative: By providing the right nutritional foundation and supporting glandular functions, any and all natural substances, including hormones, can be restored naturally.

It is easier to deal with this natural biological decline of yin when you address it early, well before menopause sets in. With appropriate diet, herbal tonics, lifestyle, exercise, and acupuncture therapy to support healthy glandular functions, you can make your passage through menopausal symptoms much smoother and actually find the journey empowering. But if you are already into menopause, these good health practices can still help you.

The Importance of Cholesterol

Cholesterol has gotten a bad rap as the agent responsible for heart disease, but cholesterol is used to produce hormones like estrogen in the body. During menopause, when hormone production slows down, cholesterol will naturally rise in the blood. That is why women at menopause and beyond find their cholesterol levels high for the first time in their lives. Besides genetic predisposition in some people, the most common causes of elevated cholesterol are poor diet and sedentary lifestyle. I'll give you suggestions here on increasing HDL, the good kind of cholesterol that protects against heart disease, while decreasing your LDL, the bad kind that contributes to plaque buildup.

Plaque formation brings about hardening of the arteries, also known as atherosclerosis. A combination of cholesterol crystals and calcium deposits, arterial plaque narrows the artery over time, impairing blood flow, and can even cause *aneurysms*, blood vessel bulges that may rupture and cause internal bleeding.

Unfortunately, because arterial plaque has no outward signs, the condition is often discovered too late, with devastating consequences. In 2004, in the United States alone, 65 percent of men and 47 percent of women with atherosclerosis experienced as their first symptom either heart attack or sudden death. One indicator in routine blood tests, called *C-reactive protein*, can alert your doctor to potential dangers. Another simple, life-saving test is the *carotid ultrasound*, which detects plaque obstructions in the arteries that supply blood to the brain. Factors that put people at higher risk for arterial plaque include diabetes, insulin intolerance, high LDL cholesterol, stress, obesity, inflammation, and high blood pressure.

Diet and emotions play a key role in high cholesterol. Chinese medicine says that cholesterol is the result of accumulated dampness and mucus due to impaired functions of the digestive system, especially that of the spleen, stomach, liver, and pancreas. This is corroborated by Western medicine, which recognizes that cholesterol is either produced by the liver or consumed in food and absorbed through the digestive tract. With natural approaches such as herbal, dietary, and exercise measures, you can reduce your blood cholesterol.

Natural Cures for Palpitations and Unsightly Veins

In menopause, due to fluctuations in arterial blood pressure and increased stress hormone levels, the heart has to work harder, pumping faster at times. Many women report that their heart races and palpitates, especially upon waking in the morning or in the middle of the night, which are frightening but, for most women, not perilous. Meditation, releasing emotional tension, and acupressure can all help reduce these episodes. However, they sometimes indicate a more dangerous condition. Researchers have found that extreme hot flashes and the corresponding palpitations are correlated with increased risk of heart disease. If heart symptoms linger, see your doctor immediately, because the incidence of heart disease in women greatly increases after menopause.

Many women also develop noticeable and sometimes painful veins in their legs that resemble twisted rope, called *varicose veins*. A milder form of this condition is known as *telangiectasia*, or *spider veins*. Varicose veins result from faulty operation of the valves within the veins that help move blood from the arms and legs back to the heart. When the valves become defective, blood pools in these veins and creates engorgement, producing bulges under the skin. Depending on their severity, they can be painful, causing a heavy sensation in the legs that is often worse at night and after exercise, ankle swelling, discoloration around the veins, and skin disorders including eczema. More common in women than men, varicose veins can be due to hereditary predisposition, pregnancy, obesity, menopause, prolonged standing, or straining associated with chronic constipation.

Varicose veins, in Chinese tradition, are due to weakness of the muscles and connective tissues of the body, which are governed by the spleen network of the digestive system. The recommendations in this chapter focus on strengthening the spleen network, supporting healthy digestive function, toning the muscles and activating movement of blood and energy. You can use acupuncture, acupressure, and massage to stimulate blood circulation and target certain veins; topical and herbal remedies will help reduce swelling and discoloration.

Don't let hot flashes make you jump out of your skin. Try to see them as moments of spiritual awakening, as surges that break through unconscious blockages, allowing emotional energy to flow again. Consider them a reminder to cultivate love, compassion, and open-heartedness. Through the wise choices you make, you will manifest the flow in your body, your mind, and ultimately your life.

The hidden meaning
of the hot flash

A hot flash sweeps over you like a storm, you feel like
you're going to explode . . . then it's gone. Soon another
one rises. But what do they mean? In Chinese tradition,
a hot flash is suppressed liver energy emerging as fire,
or unexpressed anger. So, although it is a physical
phenomenon, it brings to the surface hidden conflicts
within you. It is also a sign that you need to take time
to reevaluate your life. For the physical symptoms, soak
your feet in a hot bath, which will temporarily divert the
fire downward. Eat liver-cleansing foods and herbs such
as leafy greens, schisandra berries, ginger, rose hips, and
dandelion. Practice your qi gong. If you haven't learned
it, this is a perfect time to take a class. (If none is offered
nearby, you can learn from the DVD *Crane Style Chi Gong*
by Dr. Daoshing Ni, available at *taoofwellness.com*.) On
the spiritual level, hot flashes are telling you to take better
care of yourself, be honest with yourself, tell the truth,
and set healthy boundaries in your life.

Evening primrose for a
blossoming Second Spring

Omega-6 fatty acids are recommended by every nutritionist, physician, and health and beauty consultant these days, because these versatile substances help preserve bone health, prevent heart disease, support healthy immune functions, balance fluids, and nourish skin and hair in young and old. And for menopausal women, omega-6 fatty acids help control hot flashes. One of the richest sources of omega-6, evening primrose oil comes from the seeds of a flower that yields a bouquet of benefits. Two other natural oils, borage and black currant, are also high in omega-6 content. A typical dosage is a capsule of up to 2,000 mg of evening primrose, borage, or black currant oil daily to make one more vigorous and fend off sickness.

Soy story

Long a crucial part of the diet eaten by Okinawans, the supercentenarians of Asia, soy is packed with nutrients that are especially beneficial for women. In addition to its abundance of protein and fiber, soy is a good source of calcium, iron, potassium, B vitamins, and lecithin. And soy is rich in plant estrogen and isoflavones that alleviate hot flashes and help lower the risk of cancer, osteoporosis, and heart disease. The most potent forms of soy are the fermented types: miso, tempeh, and soy yogurt. Avoid the soy isolates found in protein powders, which can actually induce hormonal imbalance and do more harm than good. If you are among the small percentage of people who are allergic to soy, avoid it altogether as it can affect thyroid and digestive functions. But for most women, eating soy in moderation is a wonderful boon during menopause.

Keep your cool with **starflower power**

Originating in the Middle East, *starflower*, or *borage*, spread to Asia and has been incorporated for many generations into Chinese tradition as both a food and a medicine. Starflower leaves are used in salads and soups, and its beautiful star-shaped flower has a sweet, honeylike taste that is used in desserts, as a calming tea, and for ornamentation. The seed produces *borage oil*, as it is more commonly known here, the best known plant-based source of gamma linolenic acid, GLA. This omega-6 fatty acid reduces inflammation, thus helping to combat rheumatoid arthritis, nerve damage, and Alzheimer's-induced memory loss. Borage also contains oleic and palmitic acid, two fatty acids with known cholesterol-lowering properties. But the main attraction here is starflower's ability to allay hot flashes during menopause. You can make tea infusions of starflower or take the oil in supplement form, available from health food stores and Chinese herbalists.

Wild yam
can tame the flame

Your erratic, disruptive hot flashes are a direct result of hormones gone awry. Long a part of the Chinese herbal tradition, wild yam balances the body's hormonal system. It is used not only to quell hot flashes but to alleviate other menopause symptoms, such as night sweats, insomnia, and joint pain. Wild yam also strengthens the kidneys, liver, spleen, and pancreas. Studies in China have found that the fiber in Chinese wild yams helps to combat *hyperlipidemia*, a fatal disease found throughout the world, by reducing high levels of fatty lipid molecules in the bloodstream. The tuber acts to decrease insulin resistance in the body, making it an ideal food or supplement for people with diabetic tendencies. If you use whole yam, soak it before cooking. Yam extract is also available in health food stores.

Turn off the flash
with chasteberry

A traditional remedy called *chasteberry* can relieve meno-pause symptoms like hot flashes, breast tenderness, and irregular menstruation. Also called *vitex*, this herb is commonly found on riverbanks and nearby foothills in Central Asia and around the Mediterranean Sea. Research has shown that chasteberry, unlike other herbs used for women's health problems, does not contain plant estrogen or progesterone. Rather, it acts on the pituitary to stimulate balanced hormonal function, so it is also helpful in allaying PMS. Some of my patients have seen immediate relief from hot flashes within one week of taking chasteberry supplements. The usual dose is 500 to 1,000 mg daily.

Keep it down!
Blood pressure and you

Blood pressure tends to rise around menopause and even perimenopause, as estrogen in the body decreases and arteries lose elasticity. Your blood vessels constrict and your heart is stressed, pumping harder and faster. This increases the likelihood of stroke, heart and liver disease, and other problems. It can even worsen memory loss, as sustained high blood pressure inhibits proper nourishment of the brain cells. Exercise resets the tension level and stretches out the blood vessels. You can keep your blood pressure low by performing moderate physical exercise (heart rate 120 beats per minute) for half an hour to 40 minutes at least four times a week. A traditional Chinese medical remedy is to drink 8 ounces of fresh celery juice three times a day until blood pressure returns to normal. I also recommend to my patients 500 mg a day of vitamin B6, a natural diuretic; 800 mg magnesium; 1,000 mg calcium; and omega-3 supplements such as flaxseed or fish oil to provide fatty acids. Do your best to reduce your intake of things that adversely affect blood pressure: salt, caffeine, white flour, alcohol, deep-fried food, nicotine, preservatives, simple carbohydrates like sugar, and artificial flavoring and coloring. If this doesn't work within two weeks, see your physician, as high blood pressure is a condition with serious consequences.

Folic acid
to the rescue

Our bodies need amino acids for healthy metabolic function at every age, but that doesn't necessarily mean that more is better. Scientists have discovered a strong correlation between high levels of the amino acid homocysteine and loss of memory and learning ability. As you get older, your level of homocysteine rises and begins to cause inflammation, high cholesterol, and in some cases stroke or heart disease. To curb and maintain normal levels of homocysteine in the system, You can use folic acid, one of the B vitamins. Sources of folic acid include dark leafy vegetables, sunflower seeds, pumpkin seeds, peanuts, wheat germ, and liver. I suggest that my women patients in midlife take at least 800 mcg in capsule form every day.

Spring is coming—
be ready!

Research shows that as early as age 35 women begin to see changes that signal perimenopause. By age 40 many women already have decreased bone density, and irregular periods. The hot flashes may not show up until later, but if you are among those who have perimenopausal symptoms from two to ten years before the actual onset of menopause, it's important to begin to use supplements and herbs to counterbalance these changes as they occur: Vitamin B complex, especially B6 and B12, can alleviate water retention, weight gain, and mood swings. Evening primrose oil can be helpful in protecting your breasts and bones.

Acupuncture
lowers cholesterol

As you get further into your Second Spring, the hormones estrogen, progesterone, and testosterone get out of balance. Estrogen builds up the lining of the uterus and is also secreted during ovulation. Progesterone causes the lining to be eliminated during menstruation. Testosterone boosts muscle strength and libido. All three are synthesized from cholesterol. Many menopausal women see a rise in their cholesterol level that has nothing to do with diet. Why? Your body is trying to manufacture hormones as your glands decline in this function. The natural way to correct high cholesterol during menopause is to stimulate your glands to produce normal levels of hormones again. Chinese medicine relies on acupuncture and acupressure to restore healthy functioning to imbalanced organ systems. Before you take harsh cholesterol-lowering drugs and risk their side effects, see an acupuncturist. In particular, you want to work on the liver and spleen networks by stimulating the points SP-10, SP-6, and Liv-3.

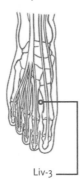

Liv-3

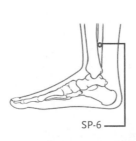

SP-6

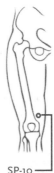

SP-10

Understanding hormone replacement therapy

For the last 30 years, Western doctors have prescribed a hormone preparation called *Prempro* for women in menopause, a combination of estrogen and progesterone from pregnant mares, hormones that the human body does not recognize. In 2002, studies concluded that women on Prempro were at elevated risk of breast cancer, uterine cancer, and heart disease, and did not gain stronger bones. The study was abruptly terminated because the risk for women clearly outweighed the benefits. For a majority of women, hormone replacement therapy (HRT) is not ideal because it shuts down the body's capability to respond to the immediate situation: Your hormonal requirements rise and fall minute by minute—your glands know this; a pill does not. Only if you have had your ovaries removed and can never manufacture enough estrogen does HRT make sense. Women who have estrogen receptor–positive breast cancer or a family history of it must avoid HRT entirely.

Artificial hormone replacement: if you do it

If your doctor offers you hormone replacement therapy as an option, it is important to know its side effects. Women taking pharmaceutical hormones who participated in the federally funded Women's Health Initiative study were found to have higher risks of breast, ovarian, and uterine cancers and well as stroke, heart attack, and blood clots. Moreover, as reported by the *New York Times*, "Most women taking the drugs did not feel more energetic, or have more sexual pleasure or even more restful sleep. The majority were not less depressed, their minds were no clearer, and their memories did not appear to have improved." Though hormone replacement therapy may still be appropriate for some as short-term therapy for menopausal distress, all the studies indicate that it should be limited to two or three years. Because of the clotting risk, do not take HRT to prevent heart disease. Its use is a personal decision, so talk to your health care provider and make an informed choice.

Natural alternatives
to artificial hormones

If you decide that hormone replacement therapy is not for you, you can turn to natural alternatives. You can prevent osteoporosis and heart disease with diet, lifestyle changes, and herbal supplement therapies. Start by making sure you eat plenty of leafy green vegetables, beans, and other foods that are rich in calcium, zinc, copper, and other minerals essential for good bone health. Fish, nuts, seeds, olives, and the oils derived from them protect you from heart disease by maintaining healthy levels of good cholesterol in your blood. Eliminating meat, cheese, and sugar from your diet will benefit not only your heart and bones, but also your waistline. Stay physically active and engage in weight-bearing, impact exercises regularly to stimulate bones and exercise your heart. Herbs such as dong quai, wild yam, and black cohosh, available from health food stores or your naturopath, can be helpful but it is important to work with experienced, licensed practitioners and nutritionists for personalized recommendations.

Estrogen overload—
it can happen to you

Advanced Western culture has developed an unfortunate phenomenon of estrogen dominance in food, medicine, and the environment. We consume dairy products from hormone-treated animals, eat plants grown with pesticides that mimic estrogen in our bodies, and use plastics, such as polychlorinated biphenyls, that also mimic estrogen. To add to all this, many women take the hormone in birth control pills. Having too much estrogen and not enough progesterone can manifest as menstrual irregularities, bloating, mood swings, acne, weight gain on the hips and abdomen, cold hands and feet, headaches, and a craving for sweets. Sound like PMS? It should—PMS produces the classic signs of estrogen-progesterone imbalance. In extreme cases, women develop PCO (polycystic ovary syndrome), in which the hormonal cycle is so out of sync that the ovarian follicles accumulate fluid but do not release an egg. To get back on track, start with exercise. Cardiovascular activities like walking, biking, aerobics, tai chi and yoga stimulate the metabolism, lower the production of follicle-stimulating hormone, and increase progesterone output.

Along came
a spider vein . . .

Varicose veins result from faulty valves within the veins that trap blood within the lower extremities, oftentimes causing throbbing pain, itching, and sometimes skin problems. In my clinical practice, I obtain very good results using acupuncture with electrical stimulation along the vein to help restore valve function. But there are many things you can do to help yourself.

First, cut out red meat and fats entirely. Avoid sugar, preservatives, artificial coloring and flavoring, salt, alcohol, and dairy. Eat lots of fresh vegetables and fruit, particularly citrus, and spices such as garlic, onions, ginger, and cayenne pepper, which contain compounds that strengthen the vein walls. Eat plenty of fish as well as omega-3 rich foods like nuts and seeds, which reduce plaque and inflammation. Eat a high-fiber lubricating diet to avoid constipation, which creates abdominal pressure and can worsen varicose veins. The herb horse chestnut, available in capsule form, can also help reduce varicose veins. Consult your acupuncturist for the proper dosage.

Chili pepper:
red hot remedy

This might be called the *miracle remedy*. The chili pepper is used traditionally in China to stimulate blood and energy flow, relieve pain, prevent the common cold, clear congestion, strengthen the immune system, reduce gas, kill parasites, and enhance stomach, brain, and kidney functions. Peppers contain a substance called *capsaicin*, which gives them their characteristic pungency and mild-to-intense heat when eaten. Capsaicin is a potent inhibitor of substance P, a neuropeptide associated with inflammatory processes. The hotter the pepper, the more capsaicin it contains. Studies indicate that chili peppers reduce blood cholesterol and triglyceride levels and decrease fibrin (which forms blood clots), thus lowering the rate of heart attack and stroke. Another benefit of the chili pepper is that its thermogenesis—the action of producing all that heat—can promote weight loss. Be warned, though: Chili peppers may exacerbate hot flashes temporarily.

Natto for a
healthy heart

In China and Japan, it is common to find fermented soybeans alongside the rice porridge and vegetables that are typical breakfast fare. This easy-to-digest food, called *natto* or *furu*, has been consumed for thousands of years for its numerous health benefits. One in particular comes in handy at midlife, when hormonal changes can affect your heart. Natto contains an enzyme called *nattokinase*, which has been shown to support heart health and promote healthy circulation. Specifically, it may dissolve *fibrin*, a protein involved in the clotting of blood; this anticoagulant action helps prevent the formation of blood clots, reducing the risk of stroke, heart attack, and deep vein thrombosis. You can take nattokinase as a supplement, but I prefer to eat the fermented soybeans—they are delicious, and a handful makes an excellent seasoning in place of salt. Consult your doctor before taking the supplement form of nattokinase if you are also taking a blood pressure medication or statin drugs, or if you will be undergoing any surgery within two weeks' time.

The PMS wake-up call

Your body is trying to get your attention. With PMS symptoms like bloating, water retention, weight gain, abdominal swelling, breast swelling, tenderness, insomnia, ravenous appetite, irritability, agitation, headaches . . . all of which may increase in intensity during perimenopause. Your body is adjusting, getting prepared for the change. Instead of an estrogen decline, you may experience an estrogen increase, another form of imbalance. Your body wants you to make adjustments in your diet and lifestyle that will serve you better in months and years to come. If you don't make those changes, when menopause comes, the symptoms will be severe.

PMS is a signal that it is time to address your deeper needs. In Chinese medicine we consider PMS a hardening of energy. We want energy to be soft, rounded, and flowing, never stagnant. But with PMS, your energy is edgy and stuck. There's a good chance you need to stop beating yourself up, be more accepting, smooth off those hard edges of self-criticism, and simply listen. Embrace your feminine energy and the symptoms will begin to ease.

A mineral that matters:
Selenium

With aging comes increased risk of heart disease and cancer, so you naturally look for help to ward them off. One of the simplest ways is to make sure your body gets enough selenium, a trace mineral used by the body to produce a potent antioxidant enzyme, glutathione peroxidase. A large-scale cancer prevention trial in 1983 demonstrated that taking a daily supplement of 200 mcg of selenium lowered the risk of developing lung, colorectal, and prostate cancer. The mineral also maintains healthy cardiovascular function by elevating the level of good cholesterol in your blood. For women in midlife, selenium has two more bonuses: It lowers your risk of joint inflammation, a common discomfort during menopause, and maintains proper glandular function by helping your body produce the most active form of thyroid hormone. Nature's powerhouse source of selenium is the Brazil nut—even a few each day can give you all you need. In supplement form, a typical dose is 100 mcg daily.

Counteract
thyroid slump

According to studies, close to 30 percent of perimeno-pausal women have low thyroid function. Once you are over 40, thyroid disease increases dramatically. But this is only part of the story. Many more women suffer from low thyroid function, but it doesn't show up on blood tests. Why? Because when estrogen is too high and is not counterbalanced by enough progesterone, this condition reduces the thyroid hormone's effectiveness in the body. So, the level may be adequate, but the thyroid hormones are not doing their work. If you have undiscovered thyroid deficiency you may feel tired all the time, gain weight for no apparent reason, or have insomnia, depression, mood swings, and brain fog; hair loss, dry skin, and constipation are also common symptoms. To get back in sync naturally, eat foods rich in iodine and minerals, such as kelp and seafood to counterbalance the estrogen by stimulating progesterone to its normal level. And detoxify your system. The liver can eliminate harmful xenoestrogens with the help of herbal cleanses, available in health food stores, which include dandelion, chrysanthemum, peppermint, and milk thistle.

Meditate for
adrenal health

Two small glands that sit atop the kidney, the *adrenals*, secrete three important hormones that help you deal with stress. The first, *epinephrine*, commonly known as *adrenaline*, helps drive blood to your heart and muscles. Most people overuse this hormone, resulting in exhaustion and malaise. *Cortisol*, the second, is a steroid that helps reduce inflammation and increase energy and appetite in traumatic and stressful situations. Too much of it can promote bone loss, kidney damage, weight gain, immune system disorders, even cancer. The third is *DHEA*, a precursor hormone that can convert into estrogen, progesterone, and testosterone. An undersupply of DHEA can lead to muscle weakness, depression, and joint pain. The adrenals help to give your body the type of hormone you need, when you need it, which is why it's so important to maintain them by regularly engaging in meditation and relaxation exercises that lower adrenaline, normalize cortisol levels, and promote abundant DHEA. Try the **Stress Release Meditation:** Breathe consciously, relax, and with each exhale focus on relaxing each area of your body in sequence, starting from the top of your head and moving down to your toes.

Nature's super-antioxidant

Grapeseed extract contains bioflavonoids called *procyanidolic oligomers* (PCOs), which are among the most powerful natural antioxidants and free radical scavengers ever discovered. Their potency is up to 50 times that of vitamin E and 20 times that of vitamin C. In your body, these strong defenders help protect and rebuild collagen to restore skin elasticity and also support the flexibility of joints and arteries. Most important, PCOs benefit the circulatory system: They enhance capillary and vein function, which helps the heart; increase peripheral circulation, which improves vision; and reduce bruising, edema from injury or trauma, varicose veins, leg swelling, and retinopathy. They cross the blood/brain barrier to protect brain tissue from oxidation. Like all antioxidants, PCOs improve immune resistance and reduce adverse allergic and inflammatory responses—but they do it bigger and better. I advise my patients that the only practical way to obtain sufficient grapeseed is by taking 100 to 200 mg a day in supplement form.

CHAPTER 8

Strengthen the Bones

MANY WOMEN GO THROUGH MENOPAUSE without any acceleration in bone loss. In fact, a number of large-scale studies, including some conducted by USDA Human Nutrition Research Center on Aging, were unsuccessful in showing a difference in bone mass in women before and after menopause. But a significant number of women have a stepped-up bone loss due to the midlife decline in estrogen, which can lead to demineralization of the bones. Certain physical consequences of menopause can take you by surprise. For example: You're walking from your car to your house with groceries, just as you have hundreds of times before. You trip over that loose stone in the walkway that you keep meaning to get fixed, but this time, instead of stumbling for a moment and perhaps cracking a couple of eggs in your grocery bag, you can't catch your balance; you fall and fracture your hip. The next thing you know, you're on your way to the hospital. How could this have happened?

When a woman fractures her hip, wrist, or other part of the skeletal structure after what seemed like an innocuous encounter with gravity, she is probably suffering from osteoporosis. Most women focus on midlife changes that affect their skin, hair, fertility, and sexuality, but osteoporosis, less obvious externally, is a serious problem that can lead to serious injuries, broken bones, lower back pain, *scoliosis* (curvature of the spine), loss of height, pain in the extremities, and even disability. The good news is that, with the right treatments and lifestyle changes, you can prevent osteoporosis and the fractured bones that result from it.

Porous Bones

It is estimated that 10 million people in the United States currently have osteoporosis, and most of them are women. In fact, while 12 percent of American men will be diagnosed with this disease, it will afflict 50 percent of American women.

Fifty percent. That's 8 to 10 times more women than men.

Additionally, one out of four women has *osteopenia*, a stage of bone loss before true osteoporosis sets in. *Osteoporosis* literally means "porous bones." Your bones are actually made of living tissue and, in a healthy person, the body constantly builds and removes bone matter, maintaining a balanced density. One kind of cell builds the bone tissue and another kind of cell removes the old tissue so it can be replaced; minerals like calcium are the currency of this exchange. Bone density peaks between the ages of 20 and 30, and thereafter begins to diminish. This reduction of bone density will continue throughout the rest of your life, though not necessarily to the point of becoming a risk to your health, and can reach 2 to 5 percent per year. Osteoporosis takes place when the cells that remove bone matter do so at a disproportionately faster rate than the cells that build it, leaving empty space in the bones, which become brittle and prone to fracture.

The cells that build bone matter in a woman's body depend heavily on the production of estrogen to function. When the onset of menopause causes estrogen production to rapidly diminish, bone building diminishes as well. While a healthy person may lose 1 percent of bone mass each year past the age of 30, nearing menopause you may lose up to 5 percent each year. A person suffering from osteoporosis may have no pain or other symptoms—perhaps a slight curvature of the spine or loss of height—until a sudden fracture occurs. That is why women at any age should take care to maintain their bone health before it is too late. Osteopenia and osteoporosis are diagnosed mainly through bone density scans of the spine, hips, and wrists. It is recommended that women begin to screen for bone health at age 35.

This chapter will help you proactively ward off bone loss with specific exercises, nutritional advice, and guidance on how to make sure your calcium supplements will be absorbed and effective.

Western Medicine and Osteoporosis

Western medicine uses four primary methods to treat osteoporosis: dietary supplementation, exercise, medication, and hormone replacement therapy. The main supplements are calcium and vitamin D, as studies have found that consuming these nutrients lowers your risk of bone fractures. Women are also advised to engage in weight-bearing exercises such as walking, working out on elliptical machines, aerobics, and resistance training with light weights to develop bone mass density and to prevent it from declining.

Some medications are effective in slowing the progress of osteoporosis but can entail various side effects ranging from inflammation to serious bone disease. One of these drugs, sodium alendronate (Fosamax), may even cause bone loss after prolonged use. Another common treatment for osteoporosis and other symptoms of menopause is hormone replacement therapy (HRT). However, as noted elsewhere in this book, HRT is associated with an increased risk of cancer, heart disease, stroke, and blood clots. It is not recommended for sustained treatment and should not be used by women with certain preexisting health problems, including migraines, liver disease, and coronary artery disease. While HRT may be effective in treating osteoporosis, there are significant questions about its overall benefit for women's health.

Medications you take for other conditions can interfere with calcium absorption and metabolism, thus affecting your bones. For example, steroids, thyroid medications, blood thinners, diuretics, and aluminum-containing drugs can deplete bone mass and speed up osteoporosis. Additionally, acid blockers and antacids can diminish calcium absorption. If you have risk factors such as a family history of osteoporosis and are taking prescription medications for any condition, be sure to discuss with your doctor alternatives that will avoid eroding your bones.

The Essence of Bones

Chinese medicine considers your essence, or *jing*, to be fundamental to the formation and maintenance of bones. Created in the kidneys, the jing does much more than form bone—it is the basis of life. A person is born with a certain amount of jing and uses it throughout life; those born with abundant amounts have a similar abundance of energy, vitality, and brain function. The seminal potency of men and the menstrual function of women depend upon the presence of jing, as well. Your essence can be drained, however, if you overindulge in food or sex, abuse drugs, or suffer from constant, unrelieved stress. If you already have a depleted level of jing by the onset of menopause, you are at heightened risk of developing conditions like osteoporosis.

This chapter provides tips on how to nurture your bones and rebuild your jing to reduce your risk of osteoporosis. Restoring your essence and vitality is a slow, deliberate process, but you can definitely do it. Here you will learn how to build the strongest bones your body can have. May you never break anything but the eggs, and may you always enjoy strength and health!

Bare-bones program to boost calcium

So many things in the typical American lifestyle deplete calcium. And when your estrogen production slows, you can lose 2 to 5 percent of bone strength per year. Here are five basic things you can do to keep your skeletal structure strong.

1) Stop smoking. You already know that tobacco adversely affects your lungs and increases your risk of cancer; it's no boon to bone health, either.

2) Eat the right kind of protein. Many American women follow diets that overload them with animal protein as a way to lose weight, which can actually leach calcium from your bones. Get your protein from vegetables and legumes such as lentils.

3) Limit salt intake. Too much can cause you to lose calcium in your urine.

4) Avoid medications that deplete calcium, including steroids, arthritis drugs, synthetic hormones, statins, and pharmaceutical antidepressants. Discuss alternatives with your naturopath or a Chinese doctor.

5) Engage in exercises that put weight on your legs: walking, running, tai chi. Bicycling will not help, but an elliptical machine at the gym will do the trick.

Are your medications bad for your bones?

When people suffer from poor digestion, their bodies are unable to digest and absorb essential nutrients. A frequent consequence, especially in older women, is a diminished capacity to maintain healthy bones. Paradoxically, some medications that are supposed to cure digestive disorders, like acid blockers for gastric reflux, present new problems for bone health. Why? Many acid-blocking medications prevent the absorption of calcium. Similarly, chemotherapy drugs, antidepressants, diuretics, steroids, and estrogen blockers all interfere with proper calcium metabolism. Be sure to talk to your doctor about the side effects of medications you are taking and how to counteract them if necessary. Better yet, if possible and if your medical doctor agrees, use natural substitutes for some pharmaceutical drugs. For example, 1 tablespoon of apple cider vinegar in a glass of water every morning on an empty stomach can ease acid reflux; St. John's wort is an excellent antidepressant; and green tea serves as a gentle diuretic.

Got greens?

Most dairy products that come from cows, such as milk and cheese, have nutritional elements that you want: calcium and protein. But when you consume cow's milk and its derivatives, there's a catch. The high protein content in dairy items acidifies the blood, causing the body to draw calcium from the bones to balance it out. The net effect of this is to leach more calcium from the body than you gain. Additionally, the protein molecules in milk are larger than the molecules a human digestive system is meant to handle, so the immune system may reject them as foreign, or allergenic. That's why many people experience fatigue, lowered ability to concentrate, and overproduction of mucus when they eat dairy. Some people lack enzymes, such as lactase, to properly digest dairy sugar; for them, consumption of dairy causes stomach pain, gas, and diarrhea. For the best protection against osteoporosis, take advantage of the absorbable calcium found in leafy greens, beans, and seeds.

Orange juice
does a body good

Calcium and vitamin D are essential for bone health. While the calcium is necessary to build and maintain bone, vitamin D is needed because the body cannot absorb calcium without it. Cow's milk has traditionally been credited as the best food for strong bones, but new studies show that your body is able to absorb both calcium and vitamin D from orange juice as readily as from milk, if not more so. (Because citrus juice's acetic acid can erode teeth enamel, don't brush your teeth for an hour after drinking juice.) Another bonus: Orange juice is full of vitamin C, a potent antioxidant that also helps facilitate calcium absorption into the body, a double benefit. So enjoy the fresh nectar of the citrus fruit while you bulk up your bones.

Sunbathe early and late— not in between

Throughout history, Chinese women have sunbathed indoors through thin rice paper screens that filter out damaging UV-A rays but admit beneficial UV-Bs. Outdoors, the women used parasols to shield their skin from the penetrating rays of the sun. Chinese tradition has always understood that sunlight is a double-edged sword. Sun is necessary for your body to produce vitamin D, essential for bone health, proper immune function, and resistance to cancer. In the West, heliotherapy is used to speed recovery from illness and treat conditions ranging from rickets to tuberculosis. But it is crucial to avoid overexposure, which can lead to premature skin aging and even cancer. To receive the benefits of sunlight, spend time outdoors before 9 a.m. and after 4 p.m. during the summer or before 10 a.m. and after 3 p.m. in winter, without sunscreen. However, if you are out in the sun in the midday hours, do use sunscreen, and if possible wear a hat and long sleeves.

Soft drinks are hard on your health

It may be satisfying to down a soft drink on a hot day—you may even feel "safe" because you're drinking the diet kind, avoiding calories so you won't put on weight. But calories aren't the only drawback in colas and other carbonated beverages—they can deplete the calcium in your bones, because they contain phosphoric acid, which makes calcium pass out of your system in the urine. Now more than ever, when you are at increased risk of osteoporosis, you want to avoid soft drinks. If you crave a bubbly refreshment, drink carbonated mineral water and add a slice of lemon!

Taking calcium supplements: how to do it right

To avoid the stooped posture and broken bones of osteo-porosis, act while you are still in your prime. Get regular weight-bearing exercise—that's smart for good health in general. But also, beginning at age 35, take proper calcium supplementation. It's not quite as easy as popping a pill, so follow these guidelines. Make sure you take calcium carbonate, the easiest type to absorb, because many forms are not really bioavailable. It must also be formulated with magnesium, preferably 1,200 mg of calcium to 600 mg of magnesium, and you will need trace amounts of boron, copper, zinc, and vitamin B3 (often included in your daily multivitamin/mineral pill). Liquid calcium in a citrate base is an excellent choice, easy to add to juice drinks or power shakes. Remember to take your calcium in several doses throughout the day, as the body cannot absorb it all at once.

The trace mineral connection to strong bones

Calcium, magnesium, and vitamin D get all the credit for maintaining good bone health, while trace minerals essential to bone formation like boron, manganese, copper, zinc, and vitamin K are often overlooked. These trace minerals act as cofactors in the bone-building process. For instance, the trace element boron positively affects the metabolism of calcium, magnesium, copper, phosphorus, and vitamin D in bone formation. Studies show that supplementation with boron reduced the loss of calcium in the urine. Boron is found in fruits, vegetables, and nuts and seeds. Vitamin K, on the other hand, found in leafy green vegetables, has been shown to be essential for specific proteins that are building blocks of bones. These are called *trace minerals* because very minute amounts of them are needed, so the supplemental dosage is very small. Daily intake of the following amounts—along with calcium, magnesium, and vitamin D—are optimal for maintaining good bone health: 10 mg boron, 5 mg manganese, 5 mg copper, 25 mg zinc, and 150 mcg vitamin K. Make sure your daily multivitamin contains these trace minerals.

Nature's boon to bones: Quercetin

Here's a lavish gift to women's health that's easy to come by—if you know what you're looking for. And from here on in, you'll want to be sure you have plenty of it. *Quercetin*, a bioflavonoid found in green tea, red wine, many plants, and microalgae, promotes the action of bone-building cells and inhibits bone resorption, or loss of minerals such as calcium. One of nature's most potent antioxidants, quercetin also supports healthy immune response, regulates estrogen balance, and acts as an anti-inflammatory. Quercetin acts on the gene that determines a cell's natural response to stress, and its presence appears to alleviate numerous kinds of pain due to inflammation, such as arthritis, allergies, fibromyalgia, and menstrual pain. Typical dosage in supplement form is 500 mg twice a day. I prefer to take microalgae as my source of quercetin, such as chlorella, blue-green algae, and spirulina, all available in health food stores. (Yes, it's good for men, too!)

Herbal help
for bone health

Chinese medicine recognizes many powerful herbs that can support bone health. *Eucommia*, used for centuries in Chinese medicine, is an important herb to encourage bone restoration. It is particularly good for back, hip, and knee pain. Eucommia helps prevent aging of the bones, and studies show that it can also increase brain function and normalize blood pressure. Other herbs that are traditionally used to help support healthy bones include black cohosh, barley grass, alfalfa, nettle, rose hips, and red clover. These herbs are brewed together as a tea to help people overcome fractures and help mend bones. It's also used before, during, and after menopause, and after labor and delivery to replenish the strength of the bones, often accompanied by soups made from large sheep or cow bones, beans and legumes, and vegetables and spices.

Caffeine without coffee:
the lift without the loss

Many people love that morning cup of coffee—it lifts the mood, jump-starts circulation, stimulates the brain, and gets the digestive system moving. The good effects of caffeine practically run the country! The bad effects, though, are especially worrisome for women at midlife and later. Too much caffeine can deplete the body's calcium just when you are at highest risk for osteoporosis, or thinning of the bone mass. If you're used to drinking coffee, now is the time to transition to green or black tea. They'll still give you caffeine but at a lower dose, and they contain vitamins, minerals, and antioxidants that help strengthen bones instead of diminishing them.

Your heels reveal the condition of your bones

A reading of the bone density in your heels can give you an idea of your bone health in other areas of your body, like your spine and hips. Tests have been approved by the FDA that measure bone density in the middle finger, heel, or shin bone. Though these localized tests are not as accurate as a full-scale bone mineral density test (BMD) like dual-energy bone densitometry (DEXA), they are useful predictors for the risk of fractures. This is especially valuable for premenopausal women and for teenage girls with eating disorders, two groups at higher risk for weak bones. A BMD test is a snapshot of your condition at a given time; for it to be useful, you must have at least two, usually one year apart, to compare the rate of mineralization or demineralization of your bones. The results are assessed in relation to normal bone density for your age. A score of 0 means you are at normal bone density for your age, minus 3 or more means osteoporosis, and a reading up to minus 2.5 means osteopenia. With proper diet, supplementation, and weight-bearing exercise, coupled with the advice given in this chapter, my patients have achieved *plus* 3 or more—signaling dramatic improvement in bone density.

Positive remodeling for net gain on your bone mass

Your bones are constantly being built up and torn down, a process called *bone remodeling*. Not unlike the upkeep on a house, your body is continually tinkering with its structure, changing its support columns on a regular basis. In an adult, up to 20 percent of bone is recycled each year. There are 206 bones in the human body, and during the growth period from childhood to adulthood, the buildup process is ahead of the tear-down process. But around the mid-30s in women (sooner if she has had pregnancies), the trend reverses, and tear-down begins to outdo buildup. Hormonal factors affect bone health. Estrogen has gotten the lion's share of attention regarding osteoporosis during menopause and beyond, but parathyroid hormone is even more directly involved in bone metabolism. The parathyroid glands sit on each side of the thyroid in the neck, and when their hormone is released in abnormally high levels, it signals the kidneys to release calcium from the bones, directly contributing to bone deterioration. Every woman over 40 should have a yearly blood test to assess thyroid and parathyroid health. If you suffer from osteopenia or osteoporosis, ask your doctor to check your parathyroid function to ensure that you are experiencing a net gain in bone mass.

Lignans from beans and
seeds for your strong bones

Instead of estrogen replacement therapy, many women are opting to increase their hormonal output the natural way, through diet, herbs, and supplementation. Beans, legumes, and seeds, for instance, contain a rich supply of lignans that are plant-source estrogens. Take your pick: black beans, kidney beans, adzuki beans, peanuts, lentils, flaxseeds, sesame seeds, and many more. Another bonus: These phytoestrogens from lignans are the good kind that will actually protect you from breast cancer.

Acupuncture pinpoints porous bones

Before you turn to prescription medications to save your bones, two natural remedies are worth a look. First, engage in weight-bearing exercise for 20 minutes, at least three or four times a week. This is your first line of defense against thinning bones. As with muscles and muscle tone, you have to use it or lose it: Work your bones and they'll stay strong. Neglect them and they'll crumble. Start walking, at least, today, and work up to longer periods of exercise. Taking supplements alone will not prevent bone loss. You have to pound the calcium into your bones with walking and other exercises that put weight on your bones.

The second prevention and treatment measure is acupuncture. Chinese medicine has been treating osteo-porosis for thousands of years with acupuncture, and in my personal practice we have seen tremendous improvement in our patients. The modern procedure, using acupuncture along with electrical stimulation, has been demonstrated to increase bone density. The method stimulates the deposit of calcium into specific bones, depending on where the needles are applied. You can also apply self-acupressure, but the use of needles elicits a more potent response.

Gravity—
it's the law

Society creates laws that dictate behavior so we can live in groups without chaos. Natural laws are a little different—we can't just vote to change them! But by learning, understanding, and applying natural laws, you can better your health. If you violate the law of gravity by deciding it doesn't apply to you and try to walk across air, you learn the consequences the hard way. Use gravity to your advantage, though, and the law is on your side. One way is to do weight-bearing exercise; gravity will strengthen your bones and help keep you free from the ravages of osteoporosis. Another way is to turn upside-down, either in yoga poses or by hanging from a bar, to increase blood flow to brain cells, relieve pressure on spinal discs, and promote circulation to the internal organs. These health benefits are available to anyone, under the law!

Get a leg up
on midlife

You have to stay strong in your Second Spring so that, after menopause, you don't become frail. To maintain the strength in your legs, perform this simple exercise. Sitting in a chair, stretch your arms out in front of you and slowly rise to a standing position. Now sit back down. Do this 10 to 15 times—and remember, keep it slow. Do this exercise at least once a day, and also incorporate a new habit into your daily activities: sit down twice! Every time you have occasion to sit in a chair, get back up and sit down again. It's easy to make this part of your routine, keeping your leg muscles strong and toned.

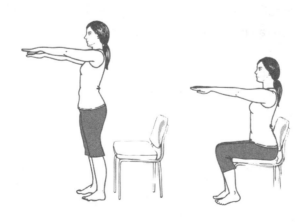

Rejuvenate growth hormones with exercise

The term *human growth hormone* usually calls up images of bodybuilders and athletes. In reality, HGH, produced by the pituitary gland in the brain, maintains healthy cell growth for everyone. When we're young, we secrete a lot of this hormone to promote bone and muscle development. After age 25, as HGH production declines, our bodies tend to have less lean tissue, more fat, and thinner skin; hair falls out, mental function wanes—all this because our cells can't replace themselves as efficiently as before. But I don't recommend artificial HGH supplementation, because the side effects can include joint discomfort and blood sugar imbalance. Instead, stimulate your body to produce more HGH on its own by performing squats to exercise the large muscles. Do leg presses at the gym; at home, simply grasp a heavy object, bend your knees, keep your spine straight, squat down and hold the position, count to 10, then come back up. In one study, squatting exercise caused an eightfold increase in HGH levels.

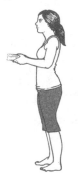
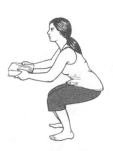

CHAPTER 9

Relieve Pain Naturally

MIDLIFE IS THE TIME when you'll notice that your body just doesn't respond to routine demands the way it used to. Maybe you're picking up your son or daughter—or a grandbaby—and you feel a stabbing pain in your shoulder, neck, or back when you straighten up. Or you mow the lawn and notice nothing unusual, only to wake up the next day feeling like a truck ran over you. Perhaps you have a mysterious ache that never seems to go away. You might not even remember when it started, or be able to locate its exact center, but you wish you didn't have to get used to it, as your medical doctor might have told you to.

When this sort of thing starts happening, the phrase "not as young as I used to be" hits home. This painful realization itself can cause you more stress, as will any worries you have about aging and going through the change—and these in turn become physical pain! That is why Chinese medicine takes a two-pronged approach to pain, using natural techniques that directly address symptoms like inflammation together with methods of alleviating emotional blockages that create or worsen pain.

In modern society, women tend to have more stress than men. The constant pressures of your job and family can lead to chronically elevated levels of the stress hormone cortisol, a direct cause of muscle and joint pain. With your busy schedule, you may neglect your own proper nutrition, living on stimulants and empty calories—does a breakfast of coffee and muffin sound familiar?—further contributing to joint pain and more generalized conditions like fibromyalgia. If you don't find time for adequate exercise, you'll develop poor circulation, the primary culprit in migraines and other headaches. Additionally, many forms of autoimmune disease, such as Sjogren's syndrome and rheumatoid arthritis, occur more during midlife and affect women more than men—nearly 79 percent of autoimmune disease patients in the United States are women. To top it all off, studies have shown that women are more sensitive to pain when they are low on estrogen, one of the classic symptoms of perimenopause.

Painkillers and Their Side Effects

As a rule, Western medicine treats pain with drugs. Whether over-the-counter or prescription, pain relief medication generally works either by reducing the inflammation at the pain site or by intervening in the area of the brain that receives pain messages. Your body in its wisdom uses pain as a wake-up call, so that you will notice, evaluate, and change the behavior that caused the pain in the first place. However, too often people simply ignore these signals from their bodies, pop a painkiller, and keep on doing whatever they are doing. This is like seeing the brake warning light of your car come on and, instead of pulling off the freeway to find out the problem, smashing the light with a hammer and driving on.

Taking a pill for pain relief, while a simple solution, makes you vulnerable to a variety of potential side effects, especially when overused: Acetaminophen (the active ingredient in Tylenol) can cause nausea and liver toxicity; ibuprofen can lead to nausea and bleeding in the gastrointestinal tract; aspirin may result in ulcers and stomach bleeding. Most narcotics, like codeine and its relative hydrocodone (found in Oxycontin and Vicodin), are addictive and can impair coordination and cognitive function while you are under their influence.

The Chinese Medicine Path to Pain Relief

Since body and mind are viewed as a parts of a whole, Chinese medicine sees pain as a symptom of energy blockage resulting from both physical and emotional imbalance. The Chinese have long recognized this multifaceted nature of pain, because pain signals through your neurons carry both physical and emotional messages. Evidence suggests that the body stores emotional trauma and memories in the connective tissues and muscles, producing unrelenting pain that cannot be alleviated by any physical medicine until the emotional trauma is released and resolved. This is why chronic pain responds effectively to the body-mind integrative approach of pain management, which includes acupuncture, meditation, and biofeedback.

While Western pain medication seeks to isolate the sensation of pain, Chinese tradition treats the underlying imbalance. For thousands of years the Chinese have been gathering knowledge about natural substances that alleviate pain. Nowadays, more and more herbs like eucommia bark and white peony root, once arcane remedies, are sold in health food stores and offered by acupuncturists and naturopaths. Both are potent agents to help quell the pain of sciatica. Other plants, like ginger and turmeric, have been employed in the West mainly as taste additives in food—in China, ginger is a traditional anti-inflammatory, administered in tea form and used in compresses placed on the pain site.

Diet is often an overlooked factor in midlife pain. Many women who suffer from arthritis find that a prescription drug treatment that works for a friend does nothing for their own pain. The Eastern model has a distinct advantage in treating arthritis. Like Western science, Chinese medicine acknowledges two main types, rheumatoid arthritis and osteoarthritis, but it breaks down the disease further, into four categories based on traditional knowledge. Depending on whether you suffer from cold, damp, heat, or wind arthritis, you will be advised to eat certain foods and avoid others. In this chapter you will learn to identify which type of arthritis you have and how you can help control it through nutrition.

Needles and Thoughts

With a history going back more than two millennia, acupuncture works by restoring the free flow of energy along the body's meridians. By freeing blockages in different circuits, acupuncture can address many common pain situations. For example, lower back pain indicates an obstruction in the kidney-bladder network, while painful joints often mean that the liver-gallbladder system is clogged. An experienced acupuncturist can, dare I say, pinpoint the treatment for your specific condition.

The mind, too, is a powerful healer that is often overlooked in strategies to alleviate pain. Visualization and meditation practices have helped many of my patients to reduce the frequency and intensity of chronic pain and even ease the recovery from traumatic injury. You don't have to reach the levels achieved by martial artists and meditating monks to make effective use of these tools in your own life. With mind-body exercises like tai chi and qi gong you can empower yourself to make your midlife transition much more comfortable.

This chapter offers a variety of tips to help you restore your body's balance and promote healthy energy flow. By taking charge of your discomfort and implementing some of these tactics and lifestyle changes, you'll have a greater opportunity to find relief from pain, and a sense of peace in knowing that you can reduce it on your own and perhaps even prevent its recurrence.

May you live happy, healthy, and in total comfort and bliss!

Soothe aches and pains with ginger

Chinese women have been using ginger to cure aches and pains for thousands of years. Inflammation is at the root of numerous ailments large and small, and ginger, the most common spice used in Chinese cooking, has been found to be a natural anti-inflammatory. It also calms nausea, inhibits bacteria such as salmonella, and increases circulation. To make ginger tea, you can either cut up the root, boil it for 10 minutes, then strain the water and sip as tea; or, if you prefer, use ginger tea bags available in health food stores. Drink it two to three times a day when you feel achy. Adding ginger when you cook—to spice up soups, for example—will also help relieve pain. For topical application, make a ginger compress: Grate the root, wrap the ginger in cheesecloth, place it in hot water for 30 seconds, then let it cool and place on the affected area for 20 minutes.

Supplements: nature's **big guns against menstrual pain and headaches**

At midlife many women still have menstrual periods, and the headache, swelling, and cramps that can go with them. Sometimes meditation and exercise are not enough to prevent or treat these pains. If you experience these problems, I recommend B-complex vitamins, not only for their pain-relieving properties but because they are crucial for energy production and specifically aid the nervous system. Vitamin B6, in particular, can be very effective for alleviating menstrual cramps, swelling, water retention, and pressure headaches. Vitamin B2, sometimes called *riboflavin*, is also quite beneficial for menstrual pain. Taking 400 mg of riboflavin and 400 mg of vitamin B6 together will be very helpful. Certain herb supplements are also powerful painkillers. Ginger, for example, fights headache and abdominal pain. You can brew the fresh root as tea—boil four slices for 10 minutes, then strain—or take one 500 mg capsule three times a day. White willow bark gives you natural *salicylic acid*, the pain-relieving ingredient in aspirin, without the stomach upset aspirin can cause. Use it for any pain you would treat with aspirin, one 500 mg capsule up to three times a day.

The Chinese herb
that masters migraines

Splitting headache? You're not alone—18 percent of American women suffer migraines, and countless others experience the less severe kind of headache. The Chinese treat these agonizing pain episodes with an herb called *Sichuan lovage*, or *ligusticum*, which has been a traditional remedy for centuries. This is a true Chinese herb, not to be confused with European lovage (levisticum). It is primarily used to provide relief from migraines and other pain conditions but also has powers to boost the immune system, activate blood circulation, and regulate menstrual periods. Studies show ligusticum's efficacy in preventing stroke and restoring blood flow to the brain and heart, and the herb has been found to inhibit tumor growth in animals. The usual dosage is 300 to 500 mg daily, or it may be taken as tea. You can find ligusticum in health food stores, online, and at the offices of acupuncturists and Chinese herbalists.

It's all in your head (and how to get it out)

Few things are as disruptive to daily life as a bad headache, especially a migraine. Medications for these debilitating episodes often don't work or cause terrible side effects. What is happening when you get a headache? In a migraine, blood vessels contract, causing pressure, inflammation, and a throbbing, pounding pain. If you have one that doesn't go away, see a doctor to rule out more serious conditions such as stroke or brain tumor. If it's a garden-variety tension headache or a migraine, you can use natural methods to relieve the pain. Diet is often the culprit: Sugar, wine, cheese, chocolate, and caffeine can all trigger or aggravate headaches (although caffeine may alleviate one temporarily, especially if you are addicted to it). Make sure you eat frequent small, nutritious meals with plenty of fruits and vegetables during the day; a supplement of B-complex vitamins can also help to reduce or prevent headaches. And, of course, stress reduction is key. Research shows that the human brain is genetically programmed to translate physical and emotional stress into headaches. Take a hot bath, get a massage, go for a walk, or meditate.

Take supplements, not shots, to ease muscle pain

When athletes get muscle pains, they tend to go to a doctor for an injection of drugs. It's no coincidence that they also tend to burn out young. There are many natural alternatives to drugs without harmful side effects. If you've already tried dietary changes, yoga, and meditation to fight muscle pain, it may be time to turn to supplements that concentrate nature's bounty for you. Muscle spasms cause a buildup in your tissues of acid that must be broken down and flushed from the system. I recommend a combination of magnesium and vitamin E. Magnesium works to counteract the acid; vitamin E promotes circulation and mops up the toxic waste. The recommended dosage is 500 mg of magnesium and 1,000 IU of vitamin E every day. *Turmeric*, a common spice found in curry, is also sold as a supplement for its anti-inflammatory properties, as research has shown its effectiveness for pain such as muscle injuries and arthritis. A typical dose is 400 mg three times a day.

Keep your
joints jumping

In herbal preparations, the bark of the eucommia tree is highly beneficial, especially in midlife, when you may experience the first creaks and twinges related to age—basically from constant use of your joints. The Chinese use this traditional remedy for back and joint pain (especially in the hips and knees) and to strengthen bones, tendons, and ligaments. Eucommia helps heal tissue that is slow to mend after an injury or that has been is weakened through stress or age. Western studies with rats confirm that both the leaves and the bark of eucommia contain a compound that encourages the development of collagen, an important part of connective tissues such as skin, tendons, and ligaments. Often used in combination with other anti-aging Chinese herbs, eucommia improves brain function and normalizes blood pressure.

What arthritis does—and
what you can do about it

If your joints have begun to trouble you, you need to be
informed about the physiology of arthritis and determine
what kind you have. *Osteoarthritis* is a simple inflammation
and degeneration of the joints. *Rheumatoid arthritis* is a
condition resulting from immune system malfunction
in which your own bodily defenses attack and erode the
joints. A natural alternative to drugs in treating osteoarthritis is supplementation with the nutrient combination
glucosamine and chondroitin. Taking at least 1,000 mg
daily can relieve pain and improve mobility. Patients with
rheumatoid arthritis have markedly reduced secretions of
interleukin-1 beta, an immune-regulating protein that helps
fight inflammation. Studies show that daily consumption
of fish oil containing a rich supply of omega-3 fatty
acids—in particular EPA and DHA—can help alleviate
joint pain and morning stiffness in rheumatoid arthritis
sufferers. To be effective, I tell my patients that the
dosage must be at least 500 mg each of EPA and DHA
on a daily basis.

Natural dietary relief for the four types of arthritis

Chinese medicine recognizes four types of arthritis: cold, wind, damp, and heat. The cold type produces sharp, stabbing, fixed pain in the joint and is exacerbated by cold and relieved by heat. Wind type manifests as pain that moves around from joint to joint and comes and goes. Damp arthritis causes dull, lingering pain in the joints or extremities, with visible swelling and persistent stiffness. In heat arthritis a sudden, acute attack makes the joint red, swollen, and warm to the touch, with pain that is relieved by cold and aggravated by heat.

We address these conditions with dietary therapy.

• **Cold arthritis** *Eat:* Warming foods such as garlic, onions, pepper, ginger, tumeric, horseradish, and anise. *Avoid:* Ice-cold beverages, dairy products.

• **Wind arthritis** *Eat:* Leafy green vegetables, grapes, black beans, whole grains, scallions. *Avoid:* Meat, shellfish, sugar, alcohol, nicotine.

• **Damp arthritis** *Eat:* Barley, millet, mung beans, mustard greens, azuki beans. *Avoid:* Dairy products, raw vegetables and fruits, ice-cold beverages. Also, do your best to avoid damp, humid environments.

• **Heat arthritis** *Eat:* Lots of raw fruits and vegetables, such as dandelion greens, cabbage, soybeans, and melons. *Avoid:* Spicy food, alcohol, tomatoes, eggplants, peppers, potatoes.

Natural oil for
creaky joints

Tiny organisms that live in the sea, *krill* are the main staple eaten by whales. Their highly nutritious oil contains high levels of *astaxanthin*, one of the most powerful antioxidants known. Astaxanthin is one of the few antioxidants that cross the blood/brain barrier, and thus may act to protect the central nervous system from free radical damage. Krill is also endowed with an unusually well-balanced fatty acid content, including not only EPA and DHA, the crucial omega-3s, but also omega-9s and phospholipids, a main structural component of living cells. Perhaps most important, clinical studies have shown that krill oil is highly effective in reducing joint discomfort in arthritis sufferers. The oil must build up in your system for full effect, so the general recommended dosage is 300 mg daily for at least a month. Make sure the product you get has been tested and proven free of harmful levels of contaminants such as mercury and other heavy metals, PCBs, and dioxins.

Stinging nettle
soothes pain

Used medicinally throughout the world for reducing inflammation, stinging nettle helps to alleviate muscular and arthritic pain. As recently as a century ago, rheumatoid arthritis sufferers would relieve pain by flogging their joints with the plant, producing a temporary stinging sensation from contact with the plant's hair and bristles. Research shows that the nettle blocks the production and action of inflammation-inducing immune cells such as cytokines and prostaglandins. It has also been used successfully to alleviate allergies, lower blood pressure, and prevent conversion of free testosterone to DHT—the culprit in many cases of hair thinning and baldness. As a temporary fix for water retention, nettle acts as a natural diuretic, reducing edema and bloating in the body. When you seek out stinging nettle supplements at your health food store, choose the right part of the plant: The root treats hair loss; the leaf fights pain, inflammation, and water retention.

No pain, no gain? Water aerobics shatters the myth!

There are natural ways to address nearly every aging symptom, but take care that the fix for one problem does not worsen another one! For example, it's common for women in their 40s to experience low energy as well as a few aches and pains. Aerobics serves as an excellent pep-up for flagging energy, but if exercise makes your pain worse, exercise in the water, which supports all your joints as you move. It is a gravity-free environment that lets you get all the cardiovascular benefit of exercise, in addition to strengthening and stretching your muscles, without hurting you. Call a nearby YWCA to see if it offers water aerobics classes, and sign up for a pain-free workout.

Scan your body
to pinpoint the pain

Sometimes you just hurt everywhere—you don't know exactly where the discomfort is coming from. When one of these generalized pain episodes strikes, you can find the source of the pain with a simple meditative practice, the body scan. Lie on your back, relax, and slow your breathing. Starting at the top of the head, with each breath focus on a small area of your body: forehead, eyes, cheeks, mouth, neck . . . concentrating your total awareness on each one in turn to discover the source of tension. Go all the way to the toes if need be, until one part lights up and tells you, "Here's your problem."

If it's your neck, stretch the muscles to ease the spasm and tightness. If it's the middle of your back, place two tennis balls on the floor a few inches apart, then lie down with your midback on top of the tennis balls and slide back and forth, allowing them to massage your muscles. (You can also put the tennis balls into a sock and tie the end to make sure they don't roll away.) These techniques will release tension and pain in many other parts of your body—once you know where to go.

Pain-free at your desk job

When you sit all day at work, your arm movements are mostly forward: writing, keyboarding, reaching across a desk. All these actions pull on your rhomboids, the muscles between your should blades, making them sore, tight, and painful. The natural way to a pain-free workday is to strengthen these muscles and keep them in shape. Two simple exercises:

1) Stand in a corner, facing the room, with one shoulder touching each wall. Take two steps forward and align your feet. With elbows bent, raise your arms to shoulder level so that your elbows contact the walls on both sides. Now use your elbows to push your chest forward, away from the wall. Inhale, push away, then exhale and lean back into the corner. Do three sets of 10 reps each, twice a day.

2) Lie face down on a bench, holding a one- or two-pound dumbbell in each hand. As you inhale, lift the dumbbells, bending your elbows, until your upper arms are parallel to the floor, squeezing your shoulder blades together. Lower your arms on the exhale. Do 10 of these twice a day.

1

2

Ergonomics for all-day energy

The human body is not made to sit in chairs or at computers all day. So we turn to the science of ergonomics, which teaches the best posture for avoiding injury and maintaining high energy.

When you sit at a desk, always have lumbar support in the lower part of your chair to help your lower back. Sit with your shoulders rolled back—slumping shoulders compress your chest cavity, causing shallow breaths, decreased oxygen to the brain, and fatigue. Your computer screen should be at eye level, so that you are looking straight ahead and not cocking your neck to see the screen. Never place the screen to the left or right of you; this will result in neck and back problems over time. The keyboard should be positioned so that your arm is at a 90-degree angle when you're typing, no higher or lower. These simple steps will ward off pain and keep you energized at work.

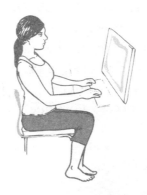

Three steps to
soothe sciatica

One of the most excruciating conditions that tends to strike at midlife is *sciatica*, an impingement of the nerve running from your lower spine down both your legs. It occurs when the sciatic nerve is compressed by muscular spasm or a herniated disc.

I treat sciatica with a three-pronged approach. First, mix the essential oils of eucalyptus, wintergreen, and camphor to make a tonic oil. Twice a day, take a 20-minute bath mixed with 2 tablespoons of tonic oil and 1 cup of Epsom salts. Second, use Chinese herbs from your health food store: White peony root helps relax muscle spasm and ease pain; peach kernel decreases swelling to alleviate the pressure; eucommia bark strengthens the lower back, bones, and tendons.

Third, acupuncture is quite effective for sciatic pain, often giving relief within a few treatments. You can also perform acupressure yourself by stimulating an acupoint called *Gallbladder-30*, located at the center of each buttock, about midway between the tip of your tailbone and the hip bone. You will naturally find an indentation that is sore. Press with your thumb (or the blunt end of a pen) and hold for 30 seconds (you will feel an achy sensation), then release. Continue for five minutes.

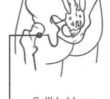

Gallbladder-30

Good point!
Acupressure eases fibromyalgia

It is estimated that 30 to 40 percent of all women develop some form of inflammatory muscle or joint condition during perimenopause and menopause. The severe form is fibromyalgia, a connective tissue disorder that often results in debilitating pain. Studies have shown that acupuncture is more effective than drug therapy in relieving the condition, and it entails no side effects. But if pain strikes when you don't have access to acupuncture, performing acupressure on yourself can be of great benefit. Work directly on the area where you are experiencing the pain. First, let your hand feel around the problem area until you locate the trigger point of the pain. When you find it, use a finger or thumb to press on the point continuously for one to two minutes, release the pressure for half a minute, then press again. Do this three times. If you can't reach the point comfortably, ask someone to help you. Often this will give you enough relief to sleep or continue your activities.

Relieve pain with healing hands—your own

Healing self-massage is a natural instinct, and you can relieve much of the pain in your body with your own hands. Here are three simple techniques. Before you begin, rub your hands together to warm them up and bring energy to your palms. The first method is to stroke the painful area with the palms flat, in a linear or circular motion, to create heat. Vigorous or gentle stroking is especially effective in the limbs.

Next is kneading. Grab your muscle between your palm and fingers and compress and pinch it as though you're kneading dough. Keep at it, squeezing and releasing—pretend you're working ingredients into an even mix. Soreness drains from muscles, tendons, ligaments, and joints, and they feel warm and relaxed.

The third technique is finger pressure, a form of acupressure. Find the most sensitive spot—wherever the pain is—and press with your thumb, or your index and middle finger together. Push down, starting with mild pressure and building to medium, then intense pressure. At the highest pressure, count to 10 as you inhale, then exhale as you release the pressure. Continue for one to three minutes.

Now, tell yourself, "Thanks, doctor!"

Stick it to your pain

Of all the midlife symptoms, pain is one of the worst obstructions to daily life. It can sap your energy, prevent you from thinking straight, and send your emotions on a downward spiral. Pharmaceutical painkillers may do their job, but they can produce dangerous side effects such as impaired cognitive function, depression, habituation—meaning your body needs more and more of the substance to produce the same result—and the very real possibility of addiction. Why not play it safe with a natural solution? Acupuncture has been found through many studies to be effective against all kinds of pain. The tiny, painless acupuncture needles stimulate the release of your body's natural painkillers, the *endorphins* and *enkephalins*. The procedure may also block the pain pathways to the brain. Work with your doctor to find the best practitioner for you, or seek referrals to an acupuncturist in your area on acupuncture.com.

Erase
your pain

That nagging pain in your back or neck—don't you wish you could just erase it? A natural method, visualization meditation, is one of the most powerful pain management tools, used with great success by pain specialists, psychologists, and biofeedback therapists. You can learn to erase pain by yourself. Here's how: Sit or lie quietly, whichever is most comfortable for you, and breathe slowly. With each exhale, feel your tension subside until you are fully relaxed. Then visualize fine vertical lines running through your body from head to toe. Keep breathing deeply as you tune in to these lines. Now bring your focus to the painful area and visualize crisscross lines at the spot that hurts. Using your imagination, erase the crisscross lines that intersect and disrupt the smooth vertical ones. Little by little, one line at a time, erase the cross-hatching with your mind until only the verticals are left. You've created a mental picture of your body's energy meridians and restored their smooth flow.

Lose a
universe of pain

The Chinese meditation exercise called *qi gong* employs
breathing, posture, and focus of the mind for healing.
Anyone can learn to relieve pain with one of its simplest
exercises: Stand with feet shoulder width apart, knees
slightly bent, and pelvis tilted forward so that your abdomen
relaxes. Keep your spine straight, shoulders pulled back
and chin tucked slightly downward. Hold your arms in
front of you as if you were cradling a basketball against
your abdomen, palms facing your torso. Take a few deep,
slow breaths and sense that your mind and body are one.
Keep your focus on the invisible ball. Now, with every
breath, imagine your body inflating and growing larger. On
the first inhale it fills up the room you're in; then exhale.
Another inhale and your body is as big as the house.
Continue: You're as big as the block, the city, the state,
the continent, the globe, until finally you're the size of

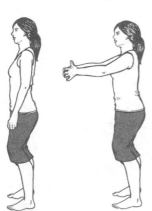

the universe. Now reverse
the process, focusing on
the exhale, with your body
shrinking in the same
sequence, from the universe
all the way back to your own
size. As you do this, you
disperse the blockage that
is causing the pain.

CHAPTER 10

Rearrange Your Home for Revitalization

YOUR HOME REPRESENTS who you are: your personality, energy, dreams, and aspirations. By its exterior colors, texture, and condition of upkeep, a house gives a feel for the person who lives there. Inside, the lighting, air, and arrangement of furniture and objects all help you refine your sense of that person subliminally. It makes no difference whether a home is small or large, an apartment or a mansion, located in the country or the city. Whatever the circumstances, your home and the conscious placement of objects within it can influence your life in a positive manner, and in turn project your best energy to the outside world.

In many ways, the magic of your Second Spring allows you to redefine who you are and who you want to be. As you experience the shift in your body, mind, and spirit during this transition, your living environment can help to shape your life the way you envision it. Ideally, what would the place you call home look, feel, smell, and sound like? When you wake up each morning, what is the first thing you want to see when you open your eyes? Would you like to surround yourself with fragrant flowers and colors that uplift your senses, or be faced with clutter that elicits agitation?

The Chinese art of feng shui is based on the science of energy alignment in one's living and work spaces to help optimize health, wealth, and happiness in one's life. You can learn how to use it for your own transformation and empowerment. I've had the good fortune to study with my father, a feng shui master who passed down to me thousands of years of wisdom about how to change people's lives through environmental alignment with positive, constructive energy. In this chapter, you will find simple yet effective suggestions for how to make your home promote personal rejuvenation, spiritual fulfillment, and physical health.

In one revealing case, I treated a patient suffering from severe indigestion who, on the advice of a gastrointestinal specialist, had taken antacids for a year without results. At first, I used a variety of traditional Chinese techniques involving diet, stress management, acupuncture, herbs, and digestive enzymes. In a few months her symptoms were reduced by about 75 percent—but they did not go away. I then turned my attention to her home environment. I learned that she had moved into her home a year earlier and still had piles of packed boxes in her living room, which was located in the middle of the house. I recognized at once that the problem was an energy blockage in her earth element, which manifests in the digestive organs. When she cleared the clutter, furnished the room comfortably, and began to inhabit it, the condition cleared up entirely.

Let It All Go . . .

The first principle for revitalizing your life through feng shui is to cleanse, detoxify, and let go of the past. If there is something you don't enjoy in your home, get rid of it to free up space and welcome in the new. Call the charity organization or have a garage sale to clear out things you haven't used or looked at in a long time. Clean your living space thoroughly to remove stains, mold, and dirt. Throw out piles of junk and any indoor plants that have died. Repair or discard broken furniture, chipped dinnerware, and cracked mirrors—these reflect aspects of your life and your health that are broken and can trap energy you need to free up and use.

. . . and Let It All Flow

The second principle of good feng shui is flow—remove blockages, smooth out rough edges and corners, and ease movement everywhere in your home. Walk around: Start with the entryway, then work your way through the living room, family room, kitchen, dining room, den, hallways, bedrooms, and bathrooms. Even the laundry area should not be overlooked. Don't forget to go to the garage and around the outside of your home. Note any furniture or fixture with sharp corners jutting out that may make you uncomfortable or block your passage. I will show how to remedy and remove blockages in your home, which reflect and even cause blockage in your life. This can mean inability to progress in your career, disconnection or miscommunication between you and your loved ones, or physical or emotional pain rooted in stifled energy.

Your Home's Light, Air, Water, and Human Energy

The third principle of correct feng shui is to fill your home with qualities that help you revitalize. Let's start with light. Our bodies cannot survive without light's energy. If you lived in constant darkness, your body would shut down, hormone output would decline, and premature aging and disease would quickly set in. Light programs the pineal gland and keeps you in sync with the circadian rhythms that govern all aspects of the body's functioning. Numerous studies have confirmed that people who are not exposed to natural light or work night shifts have higher risks of cancer, heart, and degenerative diseases. Thus, in feng shui, indoor lighting is important in dark hallways, corners of rooms, and closets. The bedroom is the only room in the house where the lighting should be dim, to promote sleep and relaxation.

The word *feng* means wind or air, and proper ventilation is key to health and well-being. It is amazing how often I walk into a home with stale, stagnant air. Nowadays, homes increasingly resemble tightly sealed boxes that trap pollution and toxins inside. Sometimes, poorly thought-out designs fail to allow for cross-ventilation, so certain areas of the home never receive fresh air. It's important to open windows regularly—even in wintertime, just a crack—to refresh the oxygen in your home. In hot areas of the country, use attic vents and fans that blow hot air out the top and draw in cool air from the ground. But as you get the air flowing, avoid drafts that blow directly on you, such as air-conditioning vents.

Water, the giver of life and sustenance, also helps move stagnant energy. At midlife women often feel stuck, unable to move forward physically and emotionally. Taking the waters for rejuvenation and relaxation has a long history in the spa traditions of Europe and Asia, and in the home the sight and sound of water helps to break up stagnant silence and move energy where it is needed. Tabletop fountains and portable waterfalls invite good energy into the house and promote healthy flow. Water is feng shui's last name—*shui* means water.

Your home environment also includes people. Your family, friends, and neighbors each possess individual energy that tends to either enrich or deplete you. Whenever it is within your control, fill your home with positive people who have uplifting energy. Help bring out the best in those you live with. When you invite toxic people into your home, after they leave you will feel ill from exposure to their energy. Make wise choices of whom you want in your home and life.

Rearranging your home for revitalization means creating a new environment conducive to your self-discovery and your new path into your Second Spring. Refresh your home, be selective, and take care of your needs. After you implement the changes I outline in this chapter, you will be pleasantly surprised by how much better you feel and the good changes that occur in your life.

Your home's immune system

In traditional Chinese households, every spring the bedding and sheets are taken outside to bake in the sun, ridding them of dampness and stale energy. Why not? It was no surprise in China when ultraviolet light was found to have sterilizing and antiseptic properties. Sunlight also stimulates the body's defense mechanisms and eliminates dampness, a factor understood to spawn pathogens. In our living and working environment, as in our bodies, dampness breeds mold and fungus that can cause allergies, tiredness, and in extreme cases, serious illness. In feng shui, the practice of energy alignment to promote health and wellness, window and door exposure to the south is favored because abundant sunlight prevents dampness and the accumulation of microbes. If your home or work environment lacks southern exposure or tends to get damp, I recommend installing an air filtration system or air purifier that uses ultraviolet technology to kill mold and fungus. Full-spectrum lightbulbs are also helpful to keep the immune system of your home or workplace in tiptop shape.

Second Spring cleaning

"Out with the old and in with the new"—this applies to both physical objects and habits of the mind at this transformational stage of life. It's time to get rid of outdated expectations and welcome your new serenity with a clear mind and a sense of openness. But this is hard to achieve in an environment cluttered with remnants of the past. Take a long hard look at all your possessions. If you've amassed magazines and catalogs, tear out and file what you want and throw the rest away. Consider which objects you can do without, and give them away or sell them—you want to make your home more spacious than it was before. If you haven't used something in a year, clothing or furniture, get rid of it. From now on, for every new thing you acquire, get rid of something else.

Unblock your door, unlock energy flow

The front door of your house or office receives energy from the world. You want it to enter easily and harmoniously, to fill and nurture your indoor environment. When you look out your door, what do you see? A closed gate, a privacy wall, your children's play structure? The worst thing for internal flow is an external blockage outside your front door. This might be any permanent object, including a tree or a telephone pole. If you do have one of these inauspicious obstacles, you may be able to remedy the situation by repositioning it—move that flagpole or utility shed to the side yard. If that's not possible, you may want to remodel to move the front door of your home or office. And if you can't do either, move! A place that does not receive abundant energy will not flourish.

Is energy slipping out your back door?

The Chinese art of feng shui has become something of a craze in certain circles, but it is often misunderstood. In the West it is often seen as a way to avoid bad energy in a site. Feng shui is the study of arranging your home and working environment to produce maximum positive energy as well. Your home should be a place of energy accumulation and proper flow. When your front door and back door face each other in a straight line, with nothing in between, you could be losing positive energy out the back door. How can you fix it? Simply put a piece of furniture somewhere in between the doors, so that you have to walk around it—ideally, a round table in the middle of the room with flowers on top. Feng shui is not just averting the negative; it's about building up positive, constructive energy.

Soften indoor edges, smooth out your life

Did you ever notice while walking down the street in a big city that when you come to intersections the wind is suddenly stronger? That's where the sharp corners of the buildings are, causing disturbance in the air flow. Similarly, sharp edges in your home can produce energy clashes that disrupt your mental flow and well-being. Look around your room. Is there a piece of furniture with sharp angles? Does it make you feel a little uncomfortable to walk by it? You want to smooth and soften indoor energy flow, and a wonderful method is to place houseplants around objects like this, sort of like energy bumpers. On the other hand, energy often stagnates in the corners of a room, getting stuck instead of circulating freely. Here too, plants are an excellent solution, bringing life and motion to these "dead spots." Water is another: Use a little decorative indoor waterfall to promote an easy, pleasant flow in your home.

Color can balance the 5 elemental energies

In feng shui, every space in the home should contain a balance of the five elements. One easy way to achieve this is to include the colors that correspond to each element. In a nutshell: Red correlates with fire and represents your passion, emotion, connection with people. Yellow is earth and corresponds to your nourishment, including intellectual. Green is wood and embodies your creativity, the ability to grow, to evolve. White is metal, representing your pure innocence and peace. Dark blue or black corresponds to water, symbolizing your faith, trust, and inner strength.

Now that you know this, you don't necessarily have to have all five colors in any given room—you can use elements instead. For example, the family room may have a round metal-framed table (metal), a festive floor lamp (fire), cushioned walnut chairs (wood), walls painted yellow (earth), and a decorative fountain (water) bubbling in one corner. Shapes also have different elemental attributes: Rooms or objects with sharp protrusions correspond to fire; square, to earth; rectangles and ovals, wood; round rooms or domed objects, metal; and meandering spaces or items, water.

Sound advice
for a calm home

Many studies have been devoted to the healing properties of sound, and you know that music you enjoy can make you feel better, whether you use it to relax or to pump up your energy. Of course, the reverse is true as well: Irritating sound can cause stress, with all its negative consequences for your health. If your home or office is routinely invaded by unwelcome sound—traffic noise, construction, or anything you find disturbing—you can counteract it by adding a subtle sound source to your environment. An indoor fountain with bubbling water calms your nerves and smoothes out your energy. Wind chimes are another option, but be sure to use the kind made from bamboo or seashells rather than metal, which can give a jangling effect. Even the sound of a grandfather clock soothes some people. Find your personal tranquilizing sound and make it the background to your day.

Within sight, within mind

The old saying "out of sight, out of mind" can actually work in reverse: The objects present in your everyday visual landscape have subtle emotional emanations that your mind absorbs. You want to fill your home with things that affect your consciousness positively. Do an inventory, look at things you take for granted—does an object or image conjure negative emotions or memories? Is a painting or artwork somehow disturbing to you? These should be replaced with bright, cheerful images that create inspiration, peace, and joy. If you are trying to get pregnant, images of happy babies—or simply words of encouragement tacked on the wall—can reinforce your intention. Here are two simple things for any interior.

1) Hang a small crystal in the window, so the dancing light it reflects will enliven the room's energy; use brightly colored glass if the space is drab.

2) Try literal images. Hang photographs of the place in the world you dream of visiting, and your subconscious spirit will subtly work to help you achieve that dream. Eliminate negativity and invite positive influences into your home, and you will see a profound influence on your life.

Don't let your money
flow down the drain

When most people think of feng shui, they think of living rooms, offices, garden paths. . . . Few pay attention to the bathroom, yet it plays a very important role in your home's energy. The counter should be clear and uncluttered, easy on the eye. A cramped room can cause energy constriction, so if your bathroom is small, use mirrors to make the space look bigger. Decorate to give a serene feeling that calms the nerves. Install a water filter to be sure you have clean water in the sink. Remember, in feng shui, water is synonymous with wealth. Fix a leaking faucet in the shower or sink immediately, and always close the toilet lid—otherwise, you are letting your wealth go down the drain!

Open the doors to life and windows to the world

We take doors and windows for granted, but to the Chinese they are symbolic: Doors represent our opening to the outside world and protection from harm; windows represent our eyes on the world, our way of connecting. In both cases, the energy flow can affect your well-being. If you live at the end of a dead-end street, too much energy will rush into the house. Create a meandering path to your door and line it with low plants. Within the hallway of a house, it is not optimal when doors to different rooms are directly opposite. Hang decorations from the ceiling to buffer the sight line between one room and another. Broken handles should be repaired immediately—every door is the door to opportunity. When you open a window, open it all the way; don't leave a small opening. (Of course, take safety measures if you have children.) Window coverings should be able to open fully, and definitely don't use shutters or blinds, which make the energy choppy. For privacy, use sheer curtains or stained or frosted glass that let in as much light as possible.

Mirror, mirror, on the wall . . .

More than just reflecting who you are, mirrors can keep energy circulating in your home. The *chi*, or universal life energy, tends to stagnate in the corners of a room, so place mirrors there to keep it flowing smoothly. You can also use mirrors to slow down an energy rush that is too intense, such as down a long hallway, by putting a mirror at the end to reflect a picture or other decoration. Don't hang a mirror in front of your bed, as it can traumatize the spirit in the middle of the night. Feng shui also uses different types of mirrors for different purposes. For example, a convex mirror deflects sharp, negative, or unwanted energy from your surroundings. If an object with sharp edges or points faces your house, it will bring unpredictable and conflicting energy into your life. Put a convex mirror above your front door to disperse it before it can enter. Always keep mirrors clean, and replace a broken one immediately.

The air you breathe
can sharpen your focus

Aromatherapy is a simple, natural way to help keep your mind alert and your energy up. Studies show that the citrus scents—lime, lemon, grapefruit, and orange—can lift your mood and increase your energy. Other pepper-upper aromas include bergamot, common herbs like basil and rosemary, lemon balm, sandalwood, and, of course, peppermint. You can turn the air you breathe into a remedy for fatigue by using incense or a natural, nonaerosol spray scent in your home. The increased focus and alertness will change everything in your day. Why not? After all, your home is *you*, at your best. When you're at work, you may want to dab the essential oil of one of these scents on your pulse points or behind your ear to sharpen your concentration.

Your bedroom, your oasis

We spend a third of our lives sleeping, so you want a nurturing environment in which to restore yourself and dream. Your bedroom is like a cocoon; it should make you feel safe and protected. First and foremost, you need a clean, uncluttered room. The bed should be placed at a diagonal to the door, but if it must be directly opposite the door, put a plant or a round table in between them. Decorate your bedroom with paired objects and symmetrical designs, because symbolically, the bedroom represents your capacity for relationships in life. You want to have pairs of pictures, for example, or two bed stands, two chairs. The bed should be raised rather than on the floor, and placed against a wall, not a window. A ringing phone is a shock to the system in the morning, so if possible, remove the phone from your bedroom. Make your bedroom a personal oasis and a sanctuary for romance.

A kitchen
to feed your soul

Without question, one of the most important rooms in the house is the kitchen. Visually, it should be decorated in one or two colors, cheery and appetizing ones. Some kitchens are long with a window at the end—this lets energy move out of the room instead of accumulating to nourish the occupants. Put a flowerpot with thriving blooms in front of the window to slow down the energy as it exits. Healthy growing things are a wonderful presence in the kitchen. Buffer the sharp edges of cabinets by hanging plants there; they will also help filter the air and counteract cooking fumes. Be sure your kitchen has a good vent to the outside, and air it out regularly by opening the windows. If you are cooking with your back toward the kitchen door, it's important to have a mirror or something reflective like a stainless steel pot in front of you, so you will see people entering. A harmonious kitchen lends positive energy to the cooking process and the food you eat.

Don't let your ceiling beam you down

In many houses, the architectural design includes exposed beams across the ceiling. This may give an artistic look to the room, but the Chinese believe, according to the principles of feng shui, that such beams disturb positive energy flow. For example, a large beam that runs across the area where you work can disrupt your personal energy; one that crosses your bedroom may even deprive you of peaceful sleep at night. That doesn't necessarily mean you have to rebuild! The solution is to drape something beautiful across the ceiling to obscure the beam, or hang plants from the beam to make it less obtrusive and soften its edges. Another solution is simply to move your couch, table, or other furniture away from the beam that is cutting off your energy.

Your indoor humidity regulator: plants

Chinese medicine has long recognized that excessive dampness or dryness can be bad for your health—dampness can create mold and other organisms that invade the lungs, and dryness harms your mucus membranes, causing respiratory problems. Either extreme is undesirable so it is important to maintain proper humidity in your house. Thousands of years ago, the Chinese discovered that certain plants act to regulate the moisture content of indoor air. Today, we have learned from scientific studies that these particular plants do a better job of balancing humidity than mechanical systems; at the same time, the plants filter out airborne toxins ranging from carbon dioxide to formaldehyde to benzene. These green regulators include bamboo, chrysanthemum, ivy, lily, and palm. Grace your home with one of these, and breathe easy.

The color of money

Students of the Chinese philosophy known as the *Tao* understand it as a practical way of life that teaches positive expressions of your being. This is also called *Living the Path of Constructive Life*, dedicated to optimum heath in body, mind, spirit, finance, and morality. Each can be cultivated through various means, including your living environment. You may be surprised to learn that your home surroundings can affect your financial health. In feng shui principles, material wealth or money correlates to the metal element, and thus can be promoted by the proper placement of metallic objects and the use of gold and silver colors in your home décor. Bronze sculptures in the foyer, a silver vase holding fresh flowers on your dining table, or a decorative waterfall placed at the western perimeter of your home so that the water flows toward the east, all bring metal elemental energies into your home. Try one or more of these to brighten your financial picture.

Grow
your own

It is a Chinese tradition to plant kumquat or orange trees on your property or in pots on your balcony, because their golden-orange fruit symbolizes wealth and prosperity. Images of fish such as koi or carp symbolize abundance, so they too are propitious in home décor. In recent years, a popular practice among feng shui aficionados is to keep a money tree in your home. A *money tree* is an indoor bonsai of the *Pachira aquatica* species. It is about one to two feet tall and bears clusters of five-lobed leaves. Take good care of the bonsai so that it radiates healthy, vibrant, and prosperous energy in your life. Of course, no matter how many money trees you have, your financial health will not improve if you don't take care of it on the functional level. You must also practice principles of good money management such as setting budgets, living within your means, and paying yourself first—always put aside money in your savings before you pay your bills. These are the ways to achieve abundance in your life.

Invite love
into your life

Second Spring is about renewal and revitalization of everything in your life, including love. If you are currently in a good relationship, take time to renew your love and be sure to keep it nurtured. If your relationship is not good, reevaluate to see if there is potential and desire for improvement. If you are not in a relationship but would like to be, the advice given here may yield surprising results. The ancient Taoist principle of five elements teaches that love emanates from the heart, which correlates with the elemental energy of fire and the color red. Take a survey of your house. Note the colors all around. Get rid of the drab ones and replace them with brighter colors in shades of red, violet, and orange. This includes wall colors, furniture, clothing, and accessories. Additionally, try to make sure that everything is in pairs. For example, replace a painting featuring one person with an image of a couple. Have two matching candlesticks instead of just one. Placing two plants of the same type in opposite corners of a room is another example of pairing. By putting emphasis on the energy of love and coupling, you will begin to attract corresponding energy into your life and find the love you deserve.

You are
where you eat

Your dining room is not just the place where you nourish your body. In feng shui it is the symbolic center of prosperity and family relationships, and the appropriate atmosphere can help them flourish. Dining room furniture should be comfortable and functional, neither too cushy nor too stark. Chairs with plump pillows tend to induce somnolence rather than relaxation here; on the other hand, furniture with austere modern lines can feel overly rigid, even unfriendly, leading to discord among the diners. An oval table is an excellent choice, or a rectangular one with rounded-off corners. There should be plenty of room for everyone to sit at the table, and clear sight lines for all. Ideally, the dining room will be a bright, open space that flows into other parts of the home. A half-wall connecting to the kitchen is one way to achieve this, or a spacious archway leading to the living room. The place where you eat should never feel isolated. These guidelines can promote healthful energy not just in your body, but in your life and among family members.

CHAPTER 11

Discover and Reinvent Your New Self

IN MANY WAYS THIS CHAPTER is the point of the entire book. Why do I want to help you to be strong, beautiful, healthy, and pain-free? So that you can come into your own in your Second Spring, fulfill your innate potential, and give the world your gift. This is your birthright and the meaning of your existence.

Youth-obsessed Western society often devalues a woman who is perceived to be past her prime and encourages her to hide or deny her age. This could not be further from the Chinese worldview. In Chinese culture, a young woman may be pretty, endearing in a way, perhaps full of potential, but true beauty comes when a woman has lived and developed character. When her face and bearing reflect the wisdom and compassion acquired by experience, a woman radiates the power of the feminine. In China, her status rises as she matures, and she is revered by her community and her family. Astonishingly to Westerners, studies have shown that the midlife transition is eagerly anticipated and produces fewer symptoms in cultures where women gain higher social status after menopause.

If you are reading this, however, most likely you live in a society where you have heard and internalized many negative attitudes about your current stage of life. This chapter is designed to help you sort out the many things you are feeling, to discard thoughts and behavior that hinder your growth, and to nurture your inherent strength and goodness. The self that you are inventing is really who you were meant to be from the start.

Suppressing Creativity Can Harm Your Body

In my practice, I have had ample opportunity to reflect on modern women's lives and the extraordinary demands placed upon them. When a woman comes to me with symptoms of exhaustion, depression, and chronic pain, these are often the side effects of neglecting the self. She may be holding down a job, raising children, managing the affairs of aging parents, constantly shouldering responsibilities for others, putting her own needs last. This syndrome is rooted in her instinctive impulse to nurture—but paradoxically, such an overload diminishes her capabilities to give and contribute. The Second Spring is a time to take a fresh, honest look at all aspects of your life and to develop new strengths. One of these is the ability to say no to demands that impinge on your health and destabilize your serenity. You can train yourself to recognize which challenges you can meet and which ones to refuse, kindly, when you cannot.

This exhilarating period in your life is also the time to manifest your inner resources in new ways. Positive impulses may end up being deflected, distorted, or suppressed in the chaos of the householding years, and their need to emerge can produce surprising phenomena. Why do so many women get fibroid tumors after age forty? Western medicine does not ask; it recommends surgery, and when the fibroids grow back, as they frequently do, more surgery. Chinese tradition recognizes these growths as physical symptoms of blocked creative energy. In other words, finding a creative outlet is more than just a metaphor! It is time to embark on your art, whatever it may be. Expressing yourself artistically does not mean aspiring to dance like Pavlova, paint like Picasso, or sing like Maria Callas. It means expressing your individuality, and it need not take the form of traditional fine arts. Many people find creative satisfaction in designing their own clothes, learning carpentry skills, revamping their home décor, or photographing events and people in their lives.

Let Freedom Flow—and Give It Your Help

Certain new freedoms come to you automatically at midlife. For example, liberated from the need for contraception after menopause, women often find that their sexuality flourishes as never before. Other freedoms require your awareness and participation. To step into your new possibilities, you will have to let go of the past—not all of it, of course, but the parts that shackle you to guilt, loss, and low self-esteem. "Easier said than done!" you may be thinking. This is true, but the task is not impossible. Many of your belief patterns are so deeply ingrained that you believe they are structural components of who you are. In this chapter, I give you specific tips on how to think about and question your past.

Typically, women fall into three destructive mindsets: comparing themselves to who they were when they were younger, dwelling on losses and traumas, and obsessing about things they wish they had done differently. Now, you are going to revitalize your energies and at the same time revise your expectations of what you can do. You will reevaluate the events in your life and, for the first time, recognize the benefits you reaped from events that traumatized you long ago. Hardest of all for some, with patient effort you can also slowly come to forgive yourself for things you have regretted for years.

Give in to Your Best Instincts

Some of the things I recommend in this chapter will surprise you. When I tell you to physically turn upside-down, it is partly to help blood flow to your brain. But I hope you will turn your life upside-down, too—out with the old, in with the new you! Toss out your old cookbooks. It's time for new recipes, guided by your tastes alone. And I'm going to ask you to throw a party for a very special guest of honor.

Try this thought exercise, especially those of you who are constantly self-critical and judgmental: Pretend for a moment that you are a newborn baby. We don't look at a baby and wish she were any different. We simply look with wonder at the way she is, taking delight in all her particulars and marveling at what she may become. This attitude is perfectly suited to your new phase of life.

Women often experience the impulse to do good deeds. This is the perfect time to fulfill these instincts, within your means, in whatever ways feel natural. You may not have room in your life for volunteer work right now, but even helping a neighbor with a task can be very gratifying. Later you may be inspired to branch out into new activities, but remember, no act of kindness is too small to enrich the world.

The first phase of your life is now the ground beneath your feet. In your Second Spring, you can be a blissful gardener, planting new growth and enjoying its fruit. May you live long and be fully yourself. The universe deserves no less.

Party
down!

You're 50—congratulations! If you have spent decades dreading this day, it's time to turn that fear around. Think back to your childhood mentality. You probably thought 50 was synonymous with ancient and decrepit. Really, don't you feel more attractive and vital at this age than you imagined you would? And things can get even better from here on. It's time to celebrate! Have a coming-out party to launch the second half of your life—call it a Second Spring celebration, and invite everyone you know. You're at a prime moment for a big life lesson: loving things as they are, including yourself.

Menopause is opportunity born out of crisis

Menopause could be called a time of crisis. In the Chinese language, *crisis* is made up of two words: *danger* and *opportunity*. The danger is that you may become mired in the past, either by having the same expectations of yourself, bemoaning your lost youth, or replaying negative scenes that you can do nothing about. But the opportunity is to change, to examine your situation with a fresh eye, to redefine *blossoming* for your Second Spring. Look at your life very honestly and you will discover new things about who you are. This is a time to grow, to explore the outside world and your inner self in ways you have not thought of before. Don't compare yourself to anyone else—relax into yourself, trust in your own joyous spirit and best instincts. You are being reborn into a wonderful second half of life.

Reawaken the spiritual centers to rejuvenate your hormones

Many spiritual traditions of the world practice some form of salutation to pay respect to a deity. In the Taoist tradition of China, salutations focus on the seven energy centers, which, not coincidentally, correlate with hormone-producing glands. At the top of the head we have the pituitary gland; between the eyes, the pineal; between the nose and lip, the hypothalamus; at the throat, the thyroid; at the midchest area, the thymus; in the stomach area, the pancreas and spleen; and in the lower abdomen, the ovaries and adrenal glands.

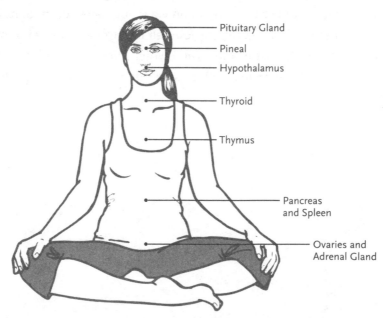

Pituitary Gland

Pineal

Hypothalamus

Thyroid

Thymus

Pancreas and Spleen

Ovaries and Adrenal Gland

Here's how to activate the seven centers in your body: In a kneeling position, raise your arms above your head until your palms touch, as though praying. Lower them until the prayer hands sit on top of your head, then form a fist with your right hand and let the left one wrap around the base of the right hand, with your thumbs pressed together. Use the first knuckle of your right middle finger to touch the seven centers one by one. Then bow forward and, keeping your hands in the same position, rest them on the ground, then touch your forehead. Repeat three times. You are stimulating your glands naturally while reconnecting body and spirit.

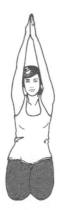 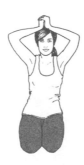 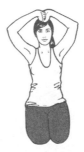

This shows how this sequence begins.

More is less: add this to your busy schedule

Most of my female patients tell me that they start their day dreading what lies ahead of them—hours of duties and exhausting demands. And they never seem to catch up on sleep. But although this may sound impossible, you need to add something to your routine: Get up a little earlier to give yourself a moment of peace first thing in the morning. Lie on the floor and stretch, sit for a while, smile, meditate on positive images. Think of the beautiful, peaceful places you've been to or hope to see someday. Envision yourself walking on the beach, hiking on a green hillside, or just relaxing by the pool. Then go for a walk, read for even a short while, or sip a cup of tea. Now, start your day from this sense of inner peace, no matter what awaits you. The mood of the day's beginning sets the tone for everything that follows.

It's your turn—
reward yourself

Women learn from early on to play the role of caretaker. After all, your body nurtures new life. The physical and emotional practice of putting someone else first soon broadens to include others besides your children. It is a beautiful form of love everyone should experience, but it often happens that others take advantage of this willingness and generosity, or you may simply take on too much, constantly deferring your own gratification. When this goes to an extreme, it can harm your emotional health. Right now, today, start planning a reward for yourself for all the things you do for others. Something that's just for you: a getaway trip, a new class, a book you've been wanting to buy . . . find that special treat that will be fulfilling and gratifying to you. Yes, ma'am, I said *you*!

Beauty is not vanity in the Second Spring

Do you feel you no longer measure up to the standards of beauty you were accustomed to earlier in life? Are you upset about the changes your body is going through? It's time to reconnect with your appreciation of your own looks. The Chinese have always recognized the resonance between inner and outer beauty: Feel it inside and it will show outside; enjoy your appearance and you will feel happier within. Now is the time to make an effort to look your best. Try a new hairstyle. Experiment with your wardrobe—wear something completely different. Even the comfort clothes you wear around the house and the sweats you take to the gym can infuse you with fresh energy. Buy new ones, feel like a new you as you embark on the second half of the wonderful journey of life. Don't forget the powerful accessory of your smile; sometimes putting on a big smile is all the makeover you need to radiate joy, health, confidence, poise, and beauty.

Don't stop asking why

Any journalist who's been trained to pursue the five W's will tell you that who, what, when, and where are simple facts to be plugged into a story—it's the why that is the crux of things. Children seem to know this instinctively, but as you get older, you just stop asking why. Yet this question is a powerful tool for finding happiness. You develop habits in life; you fall into repetitive patterns that bore you or even stop you from achieving your dreams. Start asking why again. Why do I want to be in this relationship? Why do I want to be in this job? Why do I always do this or that? Does it bring me satisfaction? Is it working? When you puzzle out these questions, you can start to do something about them. You can talk to your partner, talk to your boss, or explore new paths. With the intelligence of a journalist and the lightheartedness of a child, ask why—of others and yourself.

Now you're cooking

In active households, women can get sick of spending so much time in the kitchen. They're often expected to get up earlier than everyone else and prepare breakfast, then be ready to cook a great meal when everyone gets home from school and work—even when they themselves have jobs outside the home. They are constantly thinking about how to accommodate different people's culinary tastes and quirks. Was that your pattern? Well, this phase of life is going to be different! Now you are cooking for yourself—cooking for a new you. Give away your old cookbooks, or if they have sentimental value, store them. Replace them with new cookbooks for healthy food. Take cooking classes, collect new recipes, experiment with new ingredients. *Bon appétit!*

In the moment: a great place to live

With the pace of today's world, many people become aware of a contradiction: Your life is impossibly over-crowded, yet there is an absence, something missing. You aren't truly engaged. What is missing is the present moment. So much time is spent planning for the future, rehashing the past, wishing for something you don't have, that you never stop to really sink into what you are doing and experiencing right now. Even as you read this, you can become aware of your posture, the taste in your mouth, the air temperature, the ambient sound.... Try it. Be present in the here and now. Just notice everything around you, trying not to react judgmentally ("I wish it were cooler," "I need a better chair"). Your mind will be tempted to wander to what you'll do next or some responsibility you don't want to forget. Try to let it go and return to the present; stay focused. Most of the time we miss out on the nuances of life. Make mindfulness your new habit.

The magic word: *No*

Everyone hates disappointment—we don't like to be let down or let others down. When people ask for our help, it's natural to want to agree. But complying with every request can bring on two types of emotional discomfort. First, the work involved in fulfilling all these commitments may leave you feeling overwhelmed. And the second one can be worse: You realize that you simply can't do it all. Guilt and depression take over. You blame yourself. Now more than ever, it is time to learn to say no. Take a close look at your behavior. Do you overcommit because you feel you need to please? Or is it a habit? Whatever the reason, it's time to cut back on things you don't really want to do. Next time, before you commit, stop and be silent for a few moments. Be realistic and be honest. Can you take this on with an open heart and complete it without exhausting your energies? Learn to refuse kindly, responsibly, honestly.

You forgive others—
now try it on yourself

Centenarians are known for a common hallmark, the capacity to forgive and forget easily. When we think about that, we normally think about forgiving others. But it's even more important to forgive ourselves. In many ways, we are our own worst enemies. When we are overly self-critical and judgmental, we become paralyzed, unable to act in a positive manner, whether to move forward toward our dreams or to learn from our mistakes. Self-criticism shackles us. Accept yourself as who you are, where you are, 100 percent, even with your imperfections. Give yourself a break. Give yourself credit for your good intentions and efforts, a stroke instead of a slap. With acceptance you can begin to change, and you will be able to reach your full potential.

Good deeds
bring true happiness

Many people who live to a ripe age are naturally compassionate and serve their family and community selflessly. Everyone can learn to nurture the innate instinct to do good, even when it has been confused or covered over in the maze of conflicting messages from society. Begin to do good deeds within your means and your present circumstances, perhaps by helping out in your children's school, being a good neighbor, helping ill people, or just being a good friend. Don't force yourself—relax and do what you can. When you do good deeds or random acts of kindness, bringing happiness to those around you and bettering their lives, you are bettering the whole world, including yourself.

Make an appointment with worry—and don't come early!

One of the greatest differences between humans and our cousins the chimps is our ability to think ahead and foresee consequences. This has been a big advantage to survival, but it comes with a curse: the tendency to worry about the future. Especially at this time in your life, worries seem to accumulate, whether about concrete things like mortgages and work deadlines or more abstract matters like the challenge to remake your identity. You may spend so many waking hours consumed by anxieties that you start losing sleep. It's not easy to put worries out of your mind altogether, and in fact it's not advisable—you do need to solve those problems someday. But it helps to set aside a certain time of day to dwell on your concerns and address them. Let's say you choose 4 o'clock in the afternoon. At any other time of day, when nagging thoughts arise, you'll be able to defer them, knowing that you will take them up at the appointed time.

The unloved overachiever

Oftentimes, adult women struggle with the emotional aftereffects of not receiving enough love from their parents. They end up constantly striving for approval from their husband, their boss, or again from their parents. Such women tend to work very hard and become overachievers; they've absorbed the notion while growing up that you have to earn love instead of simply accepting it. The Superwoman Syndrome rules every aspect of their lives. This may come out as the urge to form a relationship with someone who needs to be rescued, but who is then expected to lavish Superwoman with approval and support. The syndrome creates a vicious cycle of exhaustion and resentment, in which she never gets what she wants. Examine your behavior: Does it reflect that childhood deprivation? Tell yourself that you deserve to have your needs met. Breathe deeply, and use affirmations that you create for your specific situation. You can bring about change, but only if it comes from a place of self-love and self-respect, not overcompensation.

Fibroids: symptoms of creative blockage

About 40 percent of all perimenopausal women develop fibroids in the womb, benign tumors that, if painful or bleeding, may require surgery. But in removing them, are you really taking care of the problem? In Chinese medicine we look at fibroids as manifestations of pent-up creative energy, energy that is not expressed. The uterus is an organ of procreation that nurtures new life, the most powerful organ. Fibroids are the physical manifestation of a creative force that has no outlet. Women often don't express their individuality in artistic activity because of their many obligations, caring for children, family, and so on. But if they don't address their pent-up creative energy and simply remove the symptoms, the fibroids will grow back. Start by turning to natural methods like acupuncture; avoid coffee and caffeinated drinks; meditate to allay stress; stay away from the xeno-estrogens found in plastics. Above all, you need to find creative outlets, whether writing, painting, singing, dancing—whatever you are inspired to do.

Sit with your losses, then stand tall and move on

At this time in your life, you may have gone through many losses, such as the death of parents and other griefs, perhaps when children move out on their own, perhaps in your job. The loss of reproductive ability can be another challenge, especially for women who may have dreamed of having a child but did not do so. The end of fertility, however, is not the end of everything but the beginning of a transition to the new. Allow yourself to experience it as sadness and grief, if this is how it feels to you, but know that this will not last forever, will not destroy you, and someday will be behind you. Only when you let go of the old can you move forward to welcome the new vistas and possibilities of this phase of life. You are about to explore uncharted territories and welcome newness into your life again.

Transform anger to vitality

Often, at midlife, suppressed resentment emerges as anger, either directed toward others or turned inward. In Chinese medicine, we know that anger can be transformed from a destructive force to a constructive one—vitality, energy to propel you forward, strength to make changes you may have been afraid of. Think of anger as momentum you can direct toward change. Try this exercise. Interlock your fingers in the opposite direction they would normally go: Place the backs of your hands together, interlace the fingers, and raise your hands to chest level with palms facing down, elbows straight out. Inhale first, and as you begin to exhale, pull your interlocked hands down until your arms are totally straight and your hands are pointing down. During each exhalation, blow your anger out through your breath. Repeat three to five times twice a day, or immediately after an anger episode. The more anger you have built up, the harder it will be to straighten your arms with hands firmly interlocked. As you repeat this exercise, your arms will extend more fully.

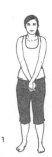

1

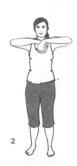

2

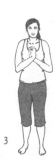

3

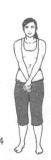

4

To stay young, hang out with youngsters

It's natural for adults to want to socialize with their own age group—and it's also natural to fall into a rut at some point. There's nothing wrong with the thought processes, topics of interest, and energy patterns of your peers, but when you make yourself available to spend time with children and adolescents, you become infected with their youthful energy. Whether you mentor younger people, teach at an after-school program, or become involved with your children's activities, exposure to the curious and adventurous mentality of the young will refresh your spirit. You'll be reminded of what you used to be like and gain new perspective on your own life. Age should not preclude nourishing the inner qualities that define youthfulness: optimism and a sense of wonderment. Go ahead and hang out with the youngsters!

Let intuition
flow

Enhanced intuition is a pleasant side effect of midlife. Hormonal changes bring about increased activity in the temporal lobe of the brain, the region associated with intuitive processes. You become wiser as you get older, not only through life experience but through the honing of the intuitive senses. Many women suppress their intuition because their culture overvalues the rational and analytical; they have no faith in their own knowing, are afraid of being wrong or humiliated for taking actions not based on reasons. The way you use your intuition will determine the way your life becomes empowered. You can use this precious gift to guide you in seeking your path. Sit quietly, try to still your intellectual mind, and start to listen to your inner voice. It can help you make the best decisions to guide the second half of your life.

Money is energy.
Are you energy
independent?

The tradition of the husband controlling family finances leaves many women in a compromised position. Money is energy, and having your own gives you self-respect and self-empowerment. Having no control over your money makes you weak and dependent.

If you're married and decide to go to Machu Picchu, fulfilling a lifelong dream, what if your husband doesn't want you to? He can refuse financial support for your trip, in effect blocking you from pursuing your dream. Of course, in a loving relationship with respect and understanding, there is mutual support, but should things go wrong, you don't want to be left powerless. It's time to gain the confidence to manage your own assets.

Women are often told that they are not good with numbers, or that they are poor money managers, but statistics show that women are better investors over the long term—they actually have superior insight into the future. The fact that women balance a household budget is widely overlooked as a skill, even by women themselves. You also have the ability to learn more sophisticated financial skills when you turn your attention to it. Learn how to invest and plan for your future and your dreams.

Age is a valuable asset

When I visit older people in assisted living facilities or meet them as my patients, I am distressed by their marginal status. Besides their physical ills, they suffer the emotional pain of abandonment by their families and society. The Chinese regard the elderly not as a liability but as a national asset, a repository of history, and a source of wisdom. The common blessing to someone in China is to wish him or her "a long and healthy life." In the United States we cast aside our experienced minds just when they are best able and ready to share their wisdom with the younger generation. If we listened to their life experience, we could continuously refine the best practices and mistakes need not be repeated by each generation. If we learn to treat our elders with respect, love, and appreciation, and provide opportunities for them to continue to contribute to society, one day we shall be treated the same way.

The midlife sandwich

Often, women in their 40s find themselves in a generational squeeze. For their teenage children, they are the adult who runs the household; for their aging parents they are the daughter in her prime who can shoulder all the details of their care. Is it humanly possible to do all this? Many women who try it end up with insomnia, anxiety, depression, and daily headaches, or even get seriously ill. Two strategies can help: building a support system and setting healthy boundaries. You may have siblings who could help and don't, or friends and neighbors who would be willing to pitch in from time to time. Tell your family members what you can do for them and what they need to do for themselves. Ask your teenager and your husband to each cook one meal per week. Have someone else care for your parents one day. Or ask to be paid! Don't wait until you get sick to set these boundaries. It won't happen overnight, but in the end everyone will benefit from the transition. Getting cancer is too big a price to pay.

An empty nest can let you spread your wings

The phrase *empty nest syndrome* was coined to describe the psychological letdown many women feel when all their children are off on their own. Now that the kids are gone, you may ask, what is my purpose? This is a wonderful opportunity to reconnect with your passions and reinvent the next half of your life. Think back to the time before the children arrived. What interests and activities did you put on hold to raise a family? What personal dreams did you have as a child or teenager? What places in the world have you always wanted to visit? Read through the journals and letters you wrote in the past and write down all the things you deferred. Assign each item a number based on its importance to you, from 1 to 5. Now think seriously about how to achieve the most important ones, and work your way down. You may be pleasantly surprised to find that this is the most personally fulfilling and evolving period of your entire life.

CHAPTER 12

Second Spring: Putting It All Together

FOR MANY WOMEN, the concept of Second Spring is a welcome, inspiring view of midlife and the changes you will go through. You may be eager to try the many tips I've given you in this book. But how, you ask yourself, will I put all this into practice? There is so much to absorb! Don't let that concern be an obstacle on your path to health and well-being. This chapter offers you a brief guide, allowing you to identify at a glance the circumstances that apply to you in your Second Spring, and get quick answers for fast relief.

Each preceding chapter gave you tools to help slow the aging process and activate your body's regenerative powers. Now, this section distills the most readily available remedies into bite-sized advice, organized by condition.

In its wisdom, Chinese medicine sees that a symptom of imbalance always has an underlying cause, and addressing it properly requires a holistic approach that takes into account your whole being—mind, body, and spirit. My approach to balance includes dietary measures, herbs and supplements, exercise, acupressure, and lifestyle factors that affect your mind and emotions. If you practice the brief meditations and other mental tips on a regular basis, you'll have satisfying results, better moods, more balance in your emotions, and greater self-awareness. Rejuvenation is not an overnight process, but if you are patient and diligent, the rewards are immense: abundant energy, inner peace, and spiritual fulfillment.

Nutrition in the Second Spring

What you eat is in some ways the most important factor in your health picture. If you are not eating a balanced diet of nutritious foods every day, you are depriving yourself of better health. The powerful compounds in good foods improve your organ functions, prevent disease, and give you energy and vitality. What you eat also affects how well you absorb the supplements you take and the nutrients in your food.

With all the dietary recommendations I make in this section, your best choice of produce is locally grown, organic, GMO-free foods in season. When you eat meat or dairy, be sure it comes from free-range, grass-fed, and hormone- and antibiotic-free animals. This helps your health and the health of the planet as well.

Herbs and Supplements

Chinese herbal medicine, one of the oldest, best-researched systems of wellness and natural healing in the world, advocates supplementing a varied diet rich in essential nutrients with additional natural substances to enhance, support, and restore your health.

It is important to take into account the fact that supplements often work in tandem with each other and with your food to benefit your health. For instance, some supplements will not be absorbed by your body without the presence of others. I highly recommend that you bring a knowledgeable wellness practitioner, such as an acupuncturist, herbalist, or naturopath, onto your health team, because an expert will be able to assess your individual needs and recommend personalized herbal and supplemental regimens. As your health strategies change and evolve, remember to also consult with your physician and, in particular, never stop taking prescription medications without your physician's input.

Exercise and Acupressure

I have never met a healthy person who was physically inactive. Regular exercise is one of your surest ways to maintain a vital metabolism. It can also alleviate hormonal swings and associated symptoms of menopause such as hot flashes, irritability, memory loss, and weight gain. Cardio-vascular exercises like bicycling, swimming, and dancing will benefit your heart health, while weight-bearing exercises like hiking or brisk walking with light weights help reduce your risk of osteoporosis. Some exercises, such as jogging and stair climbing, have both advantages.

Daily stretching or yoga helps you maintain flexibility, balance, and strength. Best of all, the mind-body exercises tai chi and qi gong are all-in-one programs that are gentle on your body but increase energy, balance organ functions, and calm your mind. To find specific exercises that address particular conditions, go to the page numbers given in this section, which refer you to more in-depth instructions in earlier chapters.

Acupuncture can treat and prevent physiological imbalances that manifest as painful or uncomfortable conditions by needles stimulating the body's energy network to get you back on track. In many instances, you can stimulate these acupoints with your own hands using acupressure. Not every single condition listed in this book has a corresponding acupoint, but where I recommend acupressure I also refer you to the illustrated page.

Lifestyle

Any time is a good time to look at your lifestyle and ask yourself whether certain habits and environments are helping or harming you. Your genetic material to some extent determines how your body will age, but a healthy lifestyle reduces the likelihood that bad genes will be expressed. Stress, for instance, is a huge factor in deteriorating health. Meditating for 15 to 20 minutes every day has numerous benefits, including reducing the output of stress hormones. Take steps to quit habits that are known to be detrimental to your health, such as smoking and excessive drinking, as these will age you before your time.

Your surroundings also play a vital role in your health and well-being. As much as possible, you want to avoid coming in contact with the toxins and chemicals that are part of our modern world. Even the subtle influence of negative people around you can affect your health. Move toward a lifestyle that is positive, uplifting, and productive, and you will be well on your way to a healthy and happy Second Spring.

Watchwords and precautions

Whenever possible, make use of the critical nutrients discussed here by incorporating their food and herb sources into your diet. If you opt to take supplements, for the most part take them with meals, since fat-soluble vitamins like vitamin E require other fats for proper absorption. Some supplements may interact with drug medications. For example, ginkgo biloba can exaggerate the anticoagulant effect of Warfarin, and garlic does the same with the platelet-inhibiting drug Tiplopidine. Vitamin C can make painkillers less effective. Always speak with your doctor before beginning a new health regimen.

Food-drug interaction can also occur, meaning that the food you eat can inhibit the medicine from working the way it should. For instance, grapefruit counteracts the cholesterol-lowering properties of statin drugs, leafy greens containing vitamin K could hinder blood thinners like Coumadin, citrus juices may decrease the efficacy of certain antibiotics, dairy products can diminish the antibacterial effect of Tetracycline, and tyramine-rich foods like alcohol and cheese interfere with antidepressants. Obviously, you should never mix alcohol with any medication or dietary supplements.

As a general rule, avoid taking prescription medication within 30 minutes of taking herbs or supplements. And don't forget to check with your doctor and pharmacist before starting any new health practice. By being well informed and working with knowledgeable health care practitioners, you can take full advantage of nature's powerful resources for your health, wellbeing and happiness.

May you live long, live strong, and live happy!

BEFORE YOU CONSIDER treating yourself with any of the following remedies, do not forget to talk to your physician. Keep in mind that the ideal way to treat any condition is to change one thing at a time: when you begin taking an herb, for example, see how it is affecting you after a week or two. Of course, you may be eager to address your health problems and want to use several remedies at once. Sometimes this is a good strategy, for example, using both acupuncture and probiotic supplements to treat certain gastrointestinal disorders. However, your best bet is to form a healing partnership that includes your Western physician along with other wellness experts such as an acupuncturist, herbalist, or naturopath. Together, they can assess your particular case and recommend the most effective combinations for you.

Arthritis / joint pain

• **Osteoarthritis,** inflammation and degeneration of the joints, can be treated with a combination of glucosamine and chondroitin. A daily dose of at least 1,000 mg of each can help relieve pain and improve mobility. *(Page 254)*

• **Rheumatoid arthritis** is an immune system malfunction in which your own bodily defenses attack and erode the joints. Fish oil—a rich source of omega-3 fatty acids, especially EPA and DHA—can help. Take every day to alleviate joint pain and morning stiffness. To be effective, I recommend to my patients that the daily dose of fish oil must contain at least 500 mg each of EPA and DHA. *(Page 254)*

• Eat the foods that help your specific type of arthritis according to Chinese precepts. *(Page 255)*

• The traditional remedy for back and joint pain is *eucommia*, which strengthens bones, tendons, and ligaments. Typical dosage is 350 mg twice a day or use the traditional Chinese Arthritis/Joint formula, which includes eucommia and other herbs. *(Page 253)*

• 300 mg of krill oil twice daily for at least a month can help to reduce joint discomfort. Make sure the product is free of harmful levels of contaminants. *(Page 256)*
• Acupuncture has been proven effective in relieving arthritic pain.

Bladder issues

• Strengthen your bladder and prevent leakage with lotus seed. Soak dried lotus seeds overnight, then use them in soups or dishes with beans or lentils. Snack on crystallized lotus seeds and add lotus paste to baked goods. Lotus seed extract is also available in powder or capsule form. The usual dose is 300 mg twice a day. *(Page 164)*
• Drinking a small cup of cranberry juice daily can help prevent bladder infections. 300 to 400 mg of cranberry in capsule form twice daily is helpful in treating an infection. *(Page 166)*
• 5,000 milligrams of vitamin C per day can help bladder infections. The recommended method is to take 1,000 mg doses every 2 or 3 hours with a cup of strong cinnamon tea, until discomfort subsides completely. This treatment may loosen bowel movement. *See your doctor if this persists beyond 3 days. (Page 165)*
• Perform kegel exercise to strengthen pelvic muscles. *(Page 163)*
• Acupuncture can strengthen the bladder sphincter and pelvic floor muscles.

Brain health (See also: Memory loss)

• For healthy brain cells, eat foods with healthy fats, such as flaxseed, almond, walnut, sesame, and olive oils, cold-water fish, nuts and seeds, avocados, and olives. *(Page 112)*
• Get a shot of brain nutrients in one natural beverage of fruit and kelp that you make in your blender. *(Page 111)*
• Sage helps improve concentration; mugwort improves delivery of nutrients to the brain; rosemary increases alertness and stimulates

brain activity. Use these brainy herbs in your cooking or brew them together as a tea and drink 3 cups per day. *(Page 115)*

• 200–400 mg of vitamin B12 daily in supplement form can help brain health. Also eat foods rich in B12: eggs, fish, and meat. *(Page 116)*

• I suggest taking 300–500 mg daily of microalgae, such as chorella, blue-green algae, spirulina, seaweed, or kelp; these are easy-to-digest, high-protein supplements that support brain vigor. *(Page 119)*

• 2 to 3 grams a day of the amino acid L-glutamine is helpful for brain health. Also, eat more L-glutamine-rich foods: beef, lamb, poultry, yogurt, raw spinach, raw parsley, and cabbage. *(Page 120)*

• Perform mental exercises to keep your cognitive functions sharp. *(Page 125)*

Digestive distress / bloating

• Eat fennel and watercress. Cut back on rich foods like dairy, meat, fats, sweets, and alcohol. *(Page 46, Page 51)*

• Avoid eating too much raw food, as it increases production of gas in the digestive system. *(Page 47)*

• Drink fluids between meals rather than with your food, so as not to dilute your gastric juices. *(Page 49)*

• Mix 1 tablespoon of organic apple cider vinegar with 12 ounces of warm water and drink in the morning on empty stomach until symptoms ease. *(Page 25)*

• Eat foods containing the dietary fiber *inulin*, which balances the helpful bacteria lining your digestive tract. Good sources include chicory root, dandelion root, Jerusalem artichoke, apples, and bananas. In supplement form, I suggest 2 grams of inulin with meals for 1 to 2 months. *(Page 97)*

Hair health

• For dry, brittle hair, eat flaxseed oil, sesame oil, olive oil, virgin coconut oil, avocado, black beans, and nuts and seeds on a regular basis. *(Page 39)*

• For shiny hair, mash a ripe avocado, massage it into your hair and scalp, and leave it on for 1 to 2 hours once per week. *(Page 38)*
• For graying hair, use *shou wu* or *fo-ti*, a hair-nurturing supplement available in Asian pharmacies. Dye your hair with natural recipes. *(Page 38)*
• Prevent hair loss by massaging your scalp with ginger juice. Leave it on overnight to stimulate the hair follicles. Typical dosage is 200 mg of an extract of stinging nettle root twice daily to treat hair loss. *(Page 38)*
• Using a natural-bristle brush, spread your hair's natural oils with full strokes from the scalp down to the tips, 100 strokes every evening. *(Page 37)*
• Every time you brush your hair, gently stroke your scalp to stimulate the hair follicles. *(Page 37)*

Headaches

• Sichuan lovage, or *ligusticum*, can provide relief from migraines. The recommended dosage is 300 to 500 mg daily as a supplement, or in tea form drink 2 or 3 cups a day. The herb is also part of the traditional Chinese formula called Headaches. *(Page 250)*
• Sugar, wine, cheese, chocolate, and caffeine can all aggravate headaches, so avoid them when one strikes or cut them out altogether if you get chronic headaches. *(Page 251)*
• Make sure you eat frequent small, nutritious meals with plenty of fruits and vegetables during the day. *(Page 251)*
• Use supplements of B-complex vitamins to alleviate pain when a headache strikes and take them daily to prevent headaches. *(Page 251)*
• Take steps to reduce stress in your life and practice a meditation technique like the **Stress Release Meditation.** *(Page 220)*
• See an acupuncturist for relief of headaches and migraines.
If you have a headache that doesn't go away, see a doctor to rule out more serious conditions, such as stroke or brain tumor.

Hearing problems

• Eat a diet rich in vitamin A and C as well as the B complex, especially niacin and folic acid: fish, carrots, citrus, asparagus, and parsley, as well as other leafy green vegetables. *(Page 129)*

• Blend 2 cloves of raw garlic and one-half an onion with 2 ounces of warm water; strain out the pulp and drink 2 ounces of the juice every day for 1 month. *(Page 129)*

• Drink a traditional Chinese tea that restores hearing function. I suggest drinking 3 times a day for 3 weeks. *(Page 130)*

• Massage your ears with traditional Chinese techniques. *(Page 133)*

Heart health

• To promote elasticity in blood vessels, take ginseng, dong quai, sacred pine, ginkgo, and hawthorn berries. Take up to 500 mg daily of each, preferably together, every day or use the traditional Chinese formula called *Super Clarity. (Page 102)*

• *Nattokinase* supports heart health and promotes healthy circulation. Eat natto (fermented soybeans) or take nattokinase as a supplement. Typical dose is 50 mg daily and the dose should contain a minimum of 1,000 FN (fibrin units). *(Page 216)*

• The mineral selenium maintains healthy cardiovascular function by elevating the level of good cholesterol in your blood. For a natural source, eat 5 or 6 Brazil nuts every day. In supplement form, consider taking 100 mcg of selenium daily. *(Page 218)*

High blood pressure (See also: Heart health)

• Limit your intake of salt, caffeine, white flour, alcohol, deep-fried food, nicotine, preservatives, sugars, and artificial flavoring and coloring. *(Page 206)*

• Drink 8 ounces of fresh celery juice 3 times a day until blood pressure returns to normal. *(Page 206)*

- I recommend 500 mg a day of vitamin B6, a natural diuretic; 800 mg of magnesium; 1,000 mg of calcium; and omega-3 supplements such as flaxseed or fish oil to provide essential fatty acids. *(Page 206)*
- Keep your blood pressure low by performing moderate exercise (heart rate 120 beats per minute) for half an hour to 40 minutes at least 4 times per week. *(Page 206)*
- Practice the **Stress Release Meditation** daily. Take your blood pressure reading before and after 15 to 20 minutes of meditation practice. Log the readings and watch your blood pressure drop over the course of a month. *(Page 220)*

If none of these remedies works within 1 month, or if your blood pressure is higher than 140 systolic and 90 diastolic, see your medical doctor immediately.

High cholesterol (See also: Heart health)

- Cut back on rich foods like dairy, meat, fats, sweets, and alcohol. *(Page 21)*
- Grate a little orange peel onto your food regularly. *(Page 29)*
- I recommend at least 800 mcg of folic acid in capsule form every day. Folic acid helps you maintain normal levels of homocysteine, which lowers cholesterol and your risk of stroke or heart disease. Sources of folic acid include dark leafy vegetables, sunflower seeds, pumpkin seeds, peanuts, wheat germ, and liver. *(Page 207)*
- Use acupuncture to correct high cholesterol. *(Page 209)*

Hot flashes

- Eat liver-cleansing foods and herbs such as leafy greens, schisandra berries, ginger, rose hips, and dandelion. *(Page 200)*
- Soy can help calm hot flashes. The fermented types of soy are most effective: miso, tempeh, natto, and soy yogurt. *(Page 202)*
- Take evening primrose oil—the richest source of omega-6—as well as borage and black currant oils. In capsule form, the typical dose is up to

2,000 mg of evening primrose, borage, or black currant oil daily. *(Page 201)*
• A daily supplement of 500 to 1,000 mg of chasteberry can help reduce hot flashes. *(Page 205)*

Insomnia
• A traditional sedative, jujube seed promotes good sleep. Recommended dosage is up to 500 mg daily as a supplement. *(Page 189)*
• Make passiflora tea by steeping 1 to 2 tablespoons of the dried herb in one cup of hot water, and drink just before bedtime. Consider taking passiflora as a supplement, 200 mg at night. *(Page 190)*
• The supplement 5-HTP has a tranquilizing effect. The recommended dosage is 200 mg at night. *(Page 191)*
• For deep relaxation, practice a breathing exercise. *(Page 192)*
• Produce a healthy relaxation response before bed, by soaking your feet in a hot bath or drinking a glass of hot soy milk with natural vanilla flavoring. *(Page 194)*
• Apply acupressure stimulation to Pericardium-6 and Kidney-1 for 10 minutes. *(Page 187)*
• Meditate or practice deep breathing for 15 minutes before bedtime. *(Page 185, Page 192)*

Low energy / fatigue
• Cut back on rich foods like dairy, meat, fats, sweets, and alcohol. *(Page 21)*
• Be sure to eat your dinner no later than 7 p.m., and eat 5 smaller meals instead of 3 large ones. *(Page 78, Page 45)*
• Eat foods that are low on the glycemic index for steady, robust energy: barley, bulgur, quinoa, amaranth, most nuts and seeds, beans and legumes, chicken, fish, and meat. *(Page 92)*
• I suggest 500 mg of magnesium per day in capsule form; consider that too much salt or dairy will interfere with absorption. Magnesium

is also found in whole grains and nuts and seeds. *(Page 79)*

• Give your system more alpha-lipoic acid. It is found in red meat, broccoli, and spinach, or you can consider taking 100 to 200 mg daily as a supplement. *(Page 82)*

• Fatigue can come from a deficiency of B vitamins. Get your B's from eggs, fish (especially shellfish), orange juice, leafy green vegetables like spinach and collard greens, and sunflower, sesame, and other seeds. Take B vitamins as a daily supplement. Be sure the product includes the whole complex and is formulated to avoid imbalance. *(Page 88)*

• For a pick-me-up, drink 2 to 3 cups of ginseng tea a day, or consider taking a daily dose of 300 mg of ginseng extract. *(Page 95)*

• Eat *black jujube date*, an energy tonic, either cooked in soup or brewed as tea. Drink 2 to 3 cups of the tea per day, using black jujube alone or combined with other energy herbs like ginseng and astragalus. *(Page 98)*

• Start a 30-minute-per-day walking routine. *(Page 89)*

• To keep your thymus healthy, take 100 to 150 mg of astragalus root per day in capsules, or drink astragalus tincture or tea 2 or 3 times a day. *(Page 86)*

• To stimulate the thymus, gently tap against the sternum (midway between the nipples) 50 times with your index and middle finger, morning and evening. *(Page 86)*

Low libido

• Eat more shellfish such as oysters, clams, mussels, shrimp, and scallops for a rich supply of zinc. Eat more pungent, spicy foods—garlic, onions, chives, cinnamon, ginger, peppers, coriander, and cardamom—to activate arousal centers. *(Page 147)*

• Argnine will boost your sex life. Arginine-rich foods include eggs and meat as well as the powerhouse sources, nuts and seeds. In supplement form, consider taking 6 to 10 grams of arginine daily. *(Page 153)*

• Get more histidine in your diet by eating more poultry, saltwater fish, meat, eggs, and soy. Take histadine as a supplement, around 500 mg a day. *(Page 155)*

• 300–450 mg horny goat weed daily can help libido enhancement. The herb is often found in supplement formulas such as Feminine Desire, along with other natural libido-boosters. *(Page 156)*

• Drink 2 cups per day of tea made from the seed of peppery daikon. Or, eat daikon in soup or salad, just like any other radish. *(Page 158)*

• I suggest 100 to 200 mg of cnidium, or snake's nest seed, about an hour before sexual activity or, to restore normal libidinal energy, daily, until improvement is seen. *(Page 159)*

Memory loss (See also: Brain health)

• To enhance cognitive ability and boost memory power, take choline supplements of up to 1,200 mg per day. Dietary sources of choline include eggs, soybeans, black beans, kidney beans, peanuts, cabbage, cauliflower, Brussels sprouts, and broccoli. *(Page 113)*

• Drink 2 to 3 cups of green tea every day. Be sure to drink it before lunch so it will not interfere with your sleep. Alternatively, decaffeinate your green tea by steeping the leaves in hot water for 1 minute, pouring out the liquid, and resteeping for 3 to 5 minutes. The amino acid L-theanine, found in green tea, benefits your mood while improving learning and concentration. In supplement form, I suggest 100 mg daily. *(Page 108, Page 121)*

• Huperzine A helps improve learning, memory retrieval, and memory retention, and may help control Alzheimer's. Its natural source is Chinese club moss (found in Asian markets); brew it as tea and drink 1 or 2 cups per day. Alternatively, I suggest 50 mcg of Huperzine A twice a day in capsule form. There are usually no side effects when the dose is kept under 100 mcg a day, but some people report gastric upset and hyperactivity when taking larger doses. *(Page 114)*

• 120 mg of ginkgo daily or drinking 2 to 3 cups of ginkgo tea every day wards off memory loss. *(Page 123)*
• Daily supplements of 2 grams of the amino acid L-carnitine can help to slow and possibly prevent memory loss. *(Page 117)*
• You can maintain a healthy memory by taking 400-500 mg of shou wu daily, or use the Chinese formula *Super Clarity*. *(Page 118)*
• Engage in cardiovascular exercise for half an hour, 5 times per week, to a heart rate of 120 beats per minute. *(Page 123)*
• Stimulate the acupressure point Kidney-3 to boost memory and concentration. *(Page 127)*

Mood swings
• Every day, eat lots of green leafy vegetables, barley grass, seaweed, anything high in chlorophyll, to keep the liver—the center of your emotions—healthy. *(Page 183)*
• 250 to 500 mg of GABA a day as a dietary supplement can help, along with 200 mg of vitamin B6, which helps your body use GABA. *(Page 179)*
• 200 mg daily of schisandra berry for a month can help calm anxiety. 500 mg dandelion daily for a month or longer can cleanse the liver and help release built-up anger. 400 mg white peony root daily for 1 to 3 months can soothe the liver and balance your mood. *(Page 184)*
• Meditate for 10 to 15 minutes when you first wake up and again before bedtime. *(Page 185)*
• Get 20 minutes of sunshine every day. *(Page 175)*
• Clear emotional blockages in your body by using massage therapy, exercise, yoga, tai chi, or qi gong to get the circuits moving. *(Page 182)*

Oseteoporosis
• Avoid smoking and do not consume soft drinks. Limit salt intake, as too much can cause calcium to be lost in your urine. Caffeine can

deplete the body's calcium. Cut out coffee and drink decaf green or black tea instead. *(Page 226, Page 231)*

• Do not take medications that deplete calcium, including steroids, arthritis drugs, synthetic hormones, statins, and pharmaceutical antidepressants. Discuss alternatives with your doctor. *(Page 227)*

• Take advantage of the absorbable calcium found in leafy greens, beans, and seeds. *(Page 228)*

• Beginning at age 35, women need to take calcium supplements. Use these guidelines for proper calcium supplementation:

At mealtime, take calcium carbonate, the easiest type to absorb, formulated with magnesium, preferably 1,200 mg of calcium to 600 mg of magnesium.

You will also need trace amounts of boron, copper, zinc, and vitamin D3 (often included in your daily multivitamin).

Liquid calcium in a citrate base is an excellent choice, easy to add to juice drinks or power shakes.

Take your calcium in several doses throughout the day, as the body cannot absorb it all at once. *(Page 232)*

• Quercetin promotes the action of bone-building cells and inhibits calcium loss. I suggest taking quercetin in supplement form, 500 mg twice a day, or get quercetin from microalgae such as chlorella, blue-green algae, and spirulina, all available in health food stores. *(Page 234)*

• Sun is necessary for your body to produce vitamin D, essential for bone health. Soak in sun by spending time outdoors before 9 a.m. and after 4 p.m. *(Page 230)*

• Engage in regular weight-bearing exercises: walking, running, tai chi. *(Page 226)*

• Acupuncture can increase bone density. See a licensed acupuncturist for treatment that stimulates the deposit of calcium into specific bones. *(Page 240)*

Sagging breasts
• Strengthen the pectoralis muscles by doing 10 push-ups a day, then work your way up to 3 sets of 10, twice a day. *(Page 30)*
• Holding a 2-pound weight in each hand, extend your arms sideways and move them in small circles, rotating toward the back. After 10 small circles, gradually widen the circles. Do 3 sets of 10 repetitions, with a little break in between, twice a day. Work your way up to 5-pound weights over time. *(Page 30)*

Skin health
• **For age-related spots and splotches,** restore your skin by restoring your kidney function. Eat a lot of black beans, sesame seeds, and mulberry. Try taking 300 mg each of Chinese yam, Asian cornelian fruit, and goji or lycium berry daily, or use an herbal formula that combines them. Consider taking supplements of 300 mg alpha-lipoic acid, 1–2 grams acetyl-L-carnitine, and 500 mg quercetin, which help skin regenerate and remove pigment deposits. *(Page 26)*
• **For dark circles under the eyes,** eat Asian or Fuji pear, which is packed with copper and vitamin C. Eat 2 of the pears daily. *(Page 23)*
• **For dry skin,** eat more flaxseed oil, sesame oil, olive oil, and virgin coconut oil. Also eat avocado and handfuls of nuts and seeds—pine nuts, hazelnuts, walnuts, sunflower seeds—on a daily basis. *(Page 39)*
• **To eliminate toxins and keep skin clear,** eat seaweed, bitter melon, Chinese cucumber, burdock, lotus root, and ginger. Use the formula Internal Cleanse, found in most Chinese herb shops. Avoid skin products containing carcinogenic chemicals. *(Page 24)*
• **For patchy, uneven skin tone,** apply organic plain yogurt like a cream to your freshly washed face, leave on for 15 minutes, then wash off with cold water. Finish up with a moisturizer. *(Page 34)*
• **To have young, healthy skin,** avoid fast food, smoking, excessive alcohol use, lack of sleep, and overexposure to sun or to dry, cold, or

windy weather. Take steps to alleviate depression, anxiety, and stress. *(See: Mood swings, page 333)* Drink at least 20 ounces of water every day. *(Page 16, Page 22)*

• Eat cherries, peanuts, black soybeans, walnuts, and jujube dates for beautiful skin. Sesame is essential for skin health. *(Page 27, Page 36)*

• I suggest taking 10–30 mg aequorin, an age-defying protein, as a daily supplement. *(Page 35)*

• **To rid the epidermis of dead skin cells on your face,** apply apple cider vinegar, diluted 2:1 with water, as a toner to your face and neck after cleansing. *(Page 25)*

• **For exfoliation,** make an herbal mask in your blender; leave it on your face for 10 minutes, scrub with a loofah, then remove with water. *(Page 20)*

• Give yourself a natural skin peel. *(Page 28)*

Vaginal dryness

• Use aloe vera with vitamin E gel for lubrication. *(Page 163)*

• Use vaginal probiotics to lubricate and soothe as well as to restore natural flora. Take pills orally or use probiotic suppositories that dissolve in the vaginal canal. You can also use plain organic yogurt as a cream. *(Page 163)*

• To restore natural lubrication and tone of vagina, consider using a teaspoon of 2% phytoestrogen cream every other day until lubrication and tone is restored. *(Page 163)*

• To increase blood flow to the area, do kegel exercises: tighten and release your vaginal muscles 10 times. *(Page 163)*

Varicose veins

• Cut out red meat and fats entirely. Avoid sugar, preservatives, artificial coloring and flavoring, salt, alcohol, and dairy. *(Page 214)*

• Be sure your diet contains lots of fresh vegetables and fruit, especially

citrus, and spices like garlic, onions, ginger, and cayenne pepper, which contain compounds that strengthen the vein walls. *(Page 214)*
• Eat plenty of fish and omega-3 rich foods like nuts and seeds, which reduce plaque and inflammation. *(Page 214)*
• A high-fiber lubricating diet is essential to avoid constipation, which creates abdominal pressure and can worsen varicose veins. *(Page 214)*
• Take the herb horse chestnut, available in capsule form. I suggest up to 600 mg daily. Consult your acupuncturist for a more precise dosage. *(Page 214)*
• Acupuncture can treat varicose veins. *(Page 214)*

Vision problems
• **For vision health,** eat at least 3 servings a day of antioxidant-rich foods such as spinach, carrots, and squash. Snack on goji berries. UV rays can damage your eyes, so wear sunglasses on bright sunny days. *(Page 135)*
• Daily supplements of 400 mg of ginkgo biloba can help improve vision. *(Page 135)*
• A Chinese remedy for clearing the eyes is to drink a juice blend of celery, peppermint, and cilantro—all rich sources of luteolin—made fresh daily. Or, I suggest 200 mg a day of luteolin in supplement form. *(Page 137)*
• **To ward off cataracts,** eat foods rich in vitamin E (spinach), vitamin C (lemons), and beta-carotene (carrots). I suggest taking daily supplements of B vitamins including 800 mg of pantothenic acid, as well as 400 IU of vitamin E, 1,000 mg or vitamin C, 10,000 IU of beta-carotene, and 150 mcg. of selenium. UV rays and nicotine both increase the risk of cataracts. Wear sunglasses and quit smoking. *(Page 138, Page 139)*
• **For tired eyes,** place slices of cucumber on your eyelids to soothe the eyes and restore moisture if they are dry. *(Page 135)*
• **To reduce floaters and maintain your vision,** practice daily eye exercises. *(Page 136)*

Weight problems

• Eat 5 small meals of healthy food every day, instead of 3 larger ones, to keep the metabolism going without storing extra reserves of fat. *(Page 45)*

• Follow these guidelines for the proper nutrition ratio in your daily diet:

25 percent animal protein: seafood, egg, chicken, turkey, and lamb (three 4-ounce portions a day).

50 percent fruits and vegetables.

25 percent divided among raw nuts and seeds, beans and legumes, and whole grains. *(Page 44)*

• Cut back on rich foods like dairy, meat, fats, sweets, and alcohol. Limit your intake of refined carbs—go for whole grains such as brown rice, whole wheat bread, quinoa, amaranth, millet, sorghum, and buckwheat. *(Page 60)*

• Eat more monounsaturated and polyunsaturated fats like vegetable, nut, and seed oils, including olive oil, rice bran oil, walnut oil, flaxseed oil, and sesame oil. Avoid trans fats at all costs. *(Page 59)*

• Instead of sugar, use the natural no-calorie herbs stevia, erythritol, and luo han guo, a fiber-filled extract called *Sweet Fiber*. *(Page 57)*

• I suggest taking conjugated linoleic acid (CLA) in supplement form, 3 to 4 grams a day. For a natural source eat beef and lamb; choose lean meat, and eat it no more than 3 times a week. *(Page 48)*

• 600 mg of NAC (N-acetyl cysteine) can help burn fat. *(Page 52)*

• Magnolia is useful for appetite control and weight management. I suggest 400 mg of magnolia as a capsule or in formulations with other herbs, or drink magnolia tea 2 to 3 times a day. *(Page 53)*

• To reverse insulin resistance, which can lead to weight gain, use cinnamon as a spice or brew it as a tea and drink 2 to 3 cups a day. *(Page 50)*

• Stimulate the acupressure point Stomach-36 to maintain a healthy metabolism. *(Page 50)*

• Perform cardio exercise 30 to 40 minutes daily. *(Page 56)*

Wrinkles

• Eat Asian or Fuji pear. This fruit is ubiquitous, from supermarkets to farmers markets. *(Page 23)*

• Tone your face with facial gymnastics. *(Page 19)*

• Perform a nonsurgical face-lift: pressing firmly with your fingers, work your way methodically along each wrinkle line, in the morning and at night. *(Page 18)*

• Consult an acupuncturist for a natural face-lift. *(Page 17)*

Resources

Ask Dr. Mao • The Natural Health Search Engine®
The official website for *Second Spring* and Dr. Mao's other books, askdrmao. com is a natural health search engine that contains thousands of searchable health questions and answers, as well as articles and blogs on health, wellness, and longevity. The health store contains selected herbal products formulated by Dr. Mao, Second Spring dietary supplements, and other health-related products, such as water filters, that are recommended by Dr. Mao.
www.askdrmao.com

Second Spring™ Health Products
Second Spring™ is a line of natural health products developed by Dr. Mao, which will benefit and rejuvenate all women. Available on secondspring.net, these products include dietary supplements, teas, drinks, and beauty products, such as Dr. Mao's regenerating cream. This Web site also features blogs, videos, and health tips for women of all ages.
www.secondspring.net

. . . .

Acupuncture and Chinese Herbal Products
Acupuncture.com is the oldest, most comprehensive, and most informative Web site on the internet for acupuncture, acupressure, Chinese herbal medicine, nutrition, tuina bodywork, tai chi, qigong, and related practices. This excellent resource for self-healing for both consumers and practitioners offers access to hundreds of publications, herbal products, and a directory of licensed practitioners throughout the United States.
www.acupuncture.com   Order line 800-772-0222

Administration on Aging
Department of Health and Human Services
For more than thirty-five years, the AOA has provided home- and community-based services to millions of seniors through the programs funded under the Older Americans Act. The AOA's Web site is full of useful information on various topics related to aging.
330 Independence Ave. SW, Suite 4760, Washington, DC 20201
www.aoa.gov   AoAInfo@aoa.hhs.gov

American Academy of Anti-Aging Medicine
An organization with a membership of 11,500 physicians and scientists from sixty-five countries, the American Academy of Anti-Aging Medicine (A4M) is

a medical society dedicated to the advancement of therapeutics related to the science of longevity medicine. Its Web site contains a wealth of research articles related to longevity and anti-aging therapeutics. It also conducts anti-aging conferences around the world.

1510 W. Montana St., Chicago, IL 60614

www.worldhealth.net   info@worldhealth.net

Arthritis Alternatives

This is an excellent resource for people suffering from arthritis. It is a Web site with a wealth of educational information on various types of arthritis and natural healing options with diet, herbs, and supplements.

www.arthritis-alternative.com

Center for Food Safety

This is a nonprofit organization fighting for strong organic standards, promoting sustainable agriculture, and protecting consumers from the hazards of pesticides and genetically engineered food.

60 Pennsylvania Ave. SE, #302 Washington, DC 20003

www.centerforfoodsafety.org   office@centerforfoodsafety.org

Center for Mind-Body Medicine

A nonprofit educational organization founded by Dr. James Gordon and dedicated to reviving the spirit and transforming the practice of medicine, the center works to create a more effective, comprehensive, and compassionate model of health care and education, combining the precision of modern science with the best of the world's healing traditions.

5225 Connecticut Ave. NW, Suite 414, Washington, DC 20015

www.cmbm.org

Chi Health Institute (CHI)

The Chi Health Institute is a non-profit association that is dedicated to promoting health and self-healing through the mind-body movement arts. The Institute offers public courses as well as professional-level education and certification programs for tai chi, qi gong, and meditation. It also maintains a directory of certified CHI instructors around the world.

www.chihealth.org

College of Tao and Integral Health

The College of Tao and Integral Health is a nonprofit, educational organization that offers distance-learning courses in Eastern health, nutrition, and dietary therapy.

Students learn at home through DVDs, CDs, and workbooks the concepts and practical healing of Eastern medicine at their own pace. This is a valuable resource for people interested in natural self-healing for themselves, as well as for those looking to become natural health educators and consultants.
www.collegeoftao.com

GNC
GNC Corporation is the nation's largest retailer of nutritional supplements offering over 5,000 retail locations throughout the United States. For store locations, go to their Web site.
www.gnc.com

Gerontology Research Group
This Web site features a group of professors, research scientists, and doctors sharing the latest findings as well as thought-provoking opinions on aging and life-extension techniques. Founded by Dr. L. Stephen Coles, MD, PhD, a professor and researcher in stem cell technology and longevity medicine at the University of California at Los Angeles School of Medicine, it also hosts monthly forums open to the public on the UCLA campus.
PO Box 905, Santa Clarita, CA 91380-9005
www.grg.org

The Grain and Salt Society
This resource offers unrefined sea salts, organic bulk whole foods, traditional cookware, hygiene products, and books.
4 Celtic Dr., Arden, NC 28704
www.celtic-seasalt.com   info@celtic-seasalt.com

Healing People Network
Healing People Network is a comprehensive Web site on the subject of complementary and alternative medicine (CAM) for consumers and practitioners. It offers in-depth coverage of subjects such as acupuncture, aromatherapy, ayurveda, bodywork, Chinese medicine, cancer risk reduction, environmental toxicology, fitness training, herbalism, homeopathy, naturopathy, nutrition and lifestyle, pet health, and other natural healing modalities. The site also provides a referral network of CAM practitioners throughout the United States and access to more than 1,000 pharmaceutical-grade supplement products.
www.healingpeople.com

Herb Research Foundation
This Web site provides useful information on well-researched therapeutic

herbs and publishes an herb magazine, *HerbalGram*.
4140 15th St., Boulder, CO 80304
www.herbs.org

Integral Living Institute
The Integral Living Institute is a nonprofit, educational organization that offers distance-learning courses and certification programs in Chinese nutrition and dietary therapy. Students learn at home through DVDs and workbooks the theories and practice of Chinese nutrition in the 3-module course at their own pace. This is a beneficial resource for people who are interested in natural self-healing for themselves, as well as for those looking to become natural health educators and consultants.
www.Integralliving.net   tot@traditionsoftao.com

National Council on Aging
Founded in 1950, the National Council on Aging is a national network of organizations and individuals dedicated to improving the health and independence of older persons and increasing their continuing contributions to communities, society, and future generations.
300 D St. SW, Suite 801, Washington, D.C. 20024
www.ncoa.gov   info@ncoa.gov

North American Menopause Society
North American Menopause Society is a nonprofit scientific organization devoted to promoting women's health and quality of life through an understanding of menopause. This site contains information on menopause, perimenopause, early menopause, menopause symptoms, and the long-term health effects of estrogen loss, as well as a wide variety of strategies and therapies to enhance health, including hormone therapy and bioidentical hormones.
www.menopause.org

Tao of Wellness
The Tao of Wellness is a health and wellness center in Southern California founded by Dr. Maoshing Ni and his brother Dr. Daoshing Ni, where they both practice with their team of associates. The center focuses on delivering exceptional treatments in acupuncture and Chinese medicine. Besides its general medicine practice, Tao of Wellness is renowned for its work in fertility, women's health, longevity, immune health, and oncology support.
1131 Wilshire Blvd., Suite 300, Santa Monica, CA 90401
www.taoofwellness.com   contact@taoofwellness.com   310-917-2200

U.S. Consumer Product Safety Commission

The CPSC's primary goals are to protect the public against unreasonable risks of injuries associated with consumer products, develop uniform safety standards, and promote research and investigation into the prevention of product-related death, injury, and illness. The commission puts out free fact sheets on hazardous products.
Washington, DC 20207
www.cpsc.gov

Vitamin Shoppe

A retail chain of more than 300 stores nationwide, it offers a large selection of vitamin and herbal supplements in store and online. For store locations, consult the Web site.
www.vitaminshoppe.com

Whole Foods Market

Founded in 1980 as one small store in Austin, Texas, Whole Foods Market is now the world's leading retailer of natural and organic foods, with more than 170 stores in North America and the United Kingdom. These stores are a good place for healthy, mostly organic food, dietary supplements, and household cleaning supplies. For store locations, consult the Web site.
525 N. Lamar, Austin, TX 78703
www.wholefoods.com

World Research Foundation

WRF established a unique, international, health information network to help people stay informed of all available treatments around the world. The nonprofit is one of the only groups that provides health information on both allopathic and alternative medicine techniques.
41 Bell Rock Plaza, Sedona, AZ 86351
www.wrf.org   info@wrf.org

Yo San University · School of Traditional Chinese Medicine

An accredited graduate school of traditional Chinese medicine founded by Dr. Maoshing Ni and his family, Yo San University's rigorous academic, clinical, and mind-body integration programs train students for the professional practice of acupuncture and Eastern medicine and carry on the Ni family medical tradition.
13315 W. Washington Blvd., Suite 200, Los Angeles, CA 90066
www.yosan.edu   admissions@yosan.edu

Index

Acknowledgments

I am indebted to my grandmother, whose life and teaching exemplified healthy expressions of feminine nature and spiritual achievement. I am grateful to my father for sharing with me her teaching in his two books, *Mystical Universal Mother* and *The Power of the Feminine*.

I am especially thankful to my patient Debbie Allen, whose own life embodies the regenerative powers of the Second Spring and who encouraged my first attempts at this book. She has been an unwavering supporter of my work for many years.

My deep appreciation to Laurie Dolphin, my untiring collaborator and partner, for her complete devotion to my writing endeavors. Her expert suggestions, designs, and illustrations have made this book much more user-friendly. She has kept this and previous projects on schedule, no small feat considering my full-time medical practice. She is living her Second Spring with pure zest!

I am indebted to Mea Argentieri for her support of my work and the generosity of her friendship. Her own transformation is a powerful testament to the possibilities for midlife revitalization. I am thankful to Helene Shaw whose personal story, as shared in media interviews, gave hope to many suffering women who later found relief through my work. I would also like to express my appreciation to Isabel Estorick for humbling me with her boundless energy, vigor, and accomplishments. All these women demonstrate the positive outcome of actualizing and living one's Second Spring.

Special thanks go to my editor at Free Press, Leslie Meredith, and to Dominick Anfuso, vice president, for their belief in my work. Leslie's thoughtful suggestions and expert editorial vision have contributed greatly to the clarity of the material. Producing a book successfully requires the efforts of many people. Much appreciation goes to Suzanne Donahue, vice president and associate publisher; Laura Davis, publishing manager; Carisa Hays, director of publicity; Shannon Gallagher, marketing manager; and the entire team at Free Press, whose collective endeavors made the book a reality. Thank you for your hard work in getting this critical information to women everywhere.

I am especially grateful to my copy editor, Elizabeth Bell, whose gift for transforming my writing into accessible and eloquent language is evidenced in this and my previous book. A special thanks to Allison Meierding for her assistance in many aspects of this book and her commitment to helping me disseminate natural healing knowledge to the world. Recognition goes to Marian Filali, who tirelessly transcribed some of my dictations, Neil Gordon for his excellent editing, and Patty Wu for her wonderful illustrations.

Thanks to Marka Meyer, the general manager of our publishing and supplement divisions and honorary house mother at Yo San University. Talk about a rejuvenated self! A grandmother, Marka can often be found running the 10k and hiking in the local hills, and never misses a beat in operating our departments and meeting the needs of all our students. Thank you for feeding me tips on the Second Spring and indulging me in my creative endeavors.

I am thankful to Stuart Shapiro, who has believed in my abilities since the early days of my professional career. Stuart is a maverick strategist whose insights into the publishing world match his extraordinary work in the political world.

My appreciation to the many patients over the years who taught me to listen and be compassionate, and who allowed me the opportunity to serve them by helping them activate the regenerative powers innate to each one.

I could not ask for a better partner in medical practice and teaching than my brother, Dr. Daoshing Ni, a women's health expert who shares the same vision for wellness medicine and has been there for me every step of the way, from the beginning of the Tao of Wellness Center to the founding of Yo San University. His wife, Sumyee Wang, who raised two boys, then went back to school and became a psychotherapist, is well on her way to experiencing an exemplary Second Spring. My deepest thanks to both of you.

Finally, I could not have completed this book without the patience and loving support of my wife, Emm, and my children, Yu-Shien Michelle, Yu-Shing Natasha, and Yu-Kai Nicholas. Thank you for everything you are, all that you do, and the sunshine you bring to my life.

May you live long, live strong and live happy!